Case No. _____

Veterinary Patient Organizer / SOAP Notebook /
History & Physical Exam Templates

By. Lance Wheeler

Property of: _____

Phone No.: _____

Date: _____

Table of Contents

Pg.	Case No.	Patient	Pg.	Case No.	Patient
104			154		
106			156		
108			158		
110			160		
112			162		
114			164		
116			166		
118			168		
120			170		
122			172		
124			174		
126			176		
128			178		
130			180		
132			182		
134			184		
136			186		
138			188		
140			190		
142			192		
144			194		
146			196		
148			198		
150			200		
152			202		

Case No._____

Patient	Age	Sex	Breed	Weight
	DOB:	Mn / Mi Fs / Fi	Color:	kg

Owner	Primary Veterinarian	Admit Date/ Time
Name: Phone:	Name: Phone:	Date: Time: AM / PM

• **Presenting Complaint**:_____
_____
_____

• **Medical Hx**:_____
_____
_____

• **When/ where obtained**:   Date:_____ ; ☐Breeder, ☐Shelter, Other:_____

Drug/ Suppl.	Amount	Dose (mg/kg)	Route	Frequency	Date Started

• **Vaccine status – Dog**: ☐Rab ☐Parv ☐Dist ☐Aden; ☐Para ☐Lep ☐Bord ☐Influ ☐Lyme
• **Vaccine status – Cat**: ☐Rab ☐Herp ☐Cali ☐Pan ☐FeLV[kittens]; ☐FIV ☐Chlam ☐Bord
• **Heartworm / Flea & Tick / Intestinal Parasites**:
    ◦ *Last Heartworm Test*: Date:_____, ☐IDK; Test Results: ☐Pos, ☐Neg, ☐IDK
    ◦ *Monthly heartworm preventative*: ☐no ☐yes, Product:_____
    ◦ *Monthly flea & tick preventative*: ☐no ☐yes, Product:_____
    ◦ *Monthly dewormer*: ☐no ☐yes, Product:_____
• **Surgical Hx**: ☐Spay/Neuter; Date:_____; Other:_____
• **Environment**: ☐Indoor, ☐Outdoor, Time spent outdoors/ Other:_____
• **Housemates**: Dogs:_____ Cats:_____ Other:_____
• **Diet**: ☐Wet, ☐Dry; Brand/ Amt.:_____

Appetite	☐Normal, ☐↑, ☐↓
Weight	☐Normal, ☐↑, ☐↓; Past Wt.:_____ kg; Date:_____; Δ:_____
Thirst	☐Normal, ☐↑, ☐↓
Urination	☐Normal, ☐↑, ☐↓, ☐Blood, ☐Strain
Defecation	☐Normal, ☐↑, ☐↓, ☐Blood, ☐Strain, ☐Diarrhea, ☐Mucus
Discharge	☐No, ☐Yes; Onset/ Describe:
Cough/ Sneeze	☐No, ☐Yes; Onset/ Describe:
Vomit	☐No, ☐Yes; Onset/ Describe:
Respiration	☐Normal, ☐↑ Rate, ☐↑ Effort
Energy level	☐Normal, ☐Lethargic, ☐Exercise intolerance

• **Travel Hx**: ☐None, Other:_____
• **Exposure to**: ☐Standing water, ☐Wildlife, ☐Board/daycare, ☐Dog park, ☐Groomer
• **Adverse reactions to food/ meds**: ☐None, Other:_____
• Can give oral meds: ☐no ☐yes; Helpful Tricks:_____

Physical Exam:

T: P: R: Wt.:   BCS: Pain: CRT:

- ☐*CV*: Regular rhythm, no murmur, normokinetic and synchronous pulses
- ☐*Resp*: Normal BV sounds/ effort, normal tracheal sounds/ palpation
- ☐*Attitude*: Bright, alert, and responsive
- ☐*Hydration/ Perfusion*: MM pink and moist with a CRT of 1-2 sec
- ☐*Eyes*: No abnormalities
- ☐*Nose*: No abnormalities
- ☐*Ears*: No abnormalities; ☐Debris (mild / mod / sev) (AU / AD / AS)
- ☐*Oral cavity*: No abnormalities; ☐Tarter (mild / mod/ sev); ☐Gingivitis
- ☐*Lymph nodes*: Small, symmetrical, smooth, and soft
- ☐*Abdomen*: Soft, non-painful, no fluid-wave, organomegaly, or masses
- ☐*Mammary Chain*: No abnormalities
- ☐*Penis/ Vulva*: No abnormalities
- ☐*Skin*: No alopecia, masses, erythema, other lesions, or ectoparasites
- ☐*Neuro*: No paresis, ataxia, or postural deficits, normal PLR and mentation
- ☐*MS*: Adequate and symmetrical muscling, no overt lameness
- ☐*Rectal*: No abnormalities, normal colored feces on glove

Labwork:

Other Diagnostics:
Blood Pressure:

Problem List:

Plan:

Case No._____

Patient	Age	Sex	Breed	Weight
	DOB:	Mn / Mi Fs / Fi	Color:	kg

Owner	Primary Veterinarian	Admit Date/ Time
Name: Phone:	Name: Phone:	Date: Time: AM / PM

• **Presenting Complaint**:_____
_____
_____

• **Medical Hx**:_____
_____
_____

• **When/ where obtained**:   Date:_____ ; □Breeder, □Shelter, Other:_____

Drug/ Suppl.	Amount	Dose (mg/kg)	Route	Frequency	Date Started

• **Vaccine status – Dog**: □Rab □Parv □Dist □Aden; □Para □Lep □Bord □Influ □Lyme
• **Vaccine status – Cat**: □Rab □Herp □Cali □Pan □FeLV[kittens]; □FIV □Chlam □Bord
• **Heartworm / Flea & Tick / Intestinal Parasites**:
   ◦ *Last Heartworm Test*: Date:_____, □IDK; Test Results: □Pos, □Neg, □IDK
   ◦ *Monthly heartworm preventative*: □no □yes, Product:_____
   ◦ *Monthly flea & tick preventative*: □no □yes, Product:_____
   ◦ *Monthly dewormer*:   □no □yes, Product:_____
• **Surgical Hx**: □Spay/Neuter; Date:_____; Other:_____
• **Environment**: □Indoor, □Outdoor, Time spent outdoors/ Other:_____
• **Housemates**: Dogs:_____ Cats:_____ Other:_____
• **Diet**: □Wet, □Dry; Brand/ Amt.:_____

Appetite	□Normal, □↑, □↓
Weight	□Normal, □↑, □↓; Past Wt.:_____ kg; Date:_____; Δ:_____
Thirst	□Normal, □↑, □↓
Urination	□Normal, □↑, □↓, □Blood, □Strain
Defecation	□Normal, □↑, □↓, □Blood, □Strain, □Diarrhea, □Mucus
Discharge	□No, □Yes; Onset/ Describe:
Cough/ Sneeze	□No, □Yes; Onset/ Describe:
Vomit	□No, □Yes; Onset/ Describe:
Respiration	□Normal, □↑ Rate, □↑ Effort
Energy level	□Normal, □Lethargic, □Exercise intolerance

• **Travel Hx**: □None, Other:_____
• **Exposure to**: □Standing water, □Wildlife, □Board/daycare, □Dog park, □Groomer
• **Adverse reactions to food/ meds**: □None, Other:_____
• Can give oral meds: □no □yes; Helpful Tricks:_____

Physical Exam:

T: *P:*   *R:*   *Wt.:*   *BCS:*   *Pain:*   *CRT:*

☐*CV*: Regular rhythm, no murmur, normokinetic and synchronous pulses
☐*Resp*: Normal BV sounds/ effort, normal tracheal sounds/ palpation
☐*Attitude*: Bright, alert, and responsive
☐*Hydration/ Perfusion*: MM pink and moist with a CRT of 1-2 sec
☐*Eyes*: No abnormalities
☐*Nose*: No abnormalities
☐*Ears*: No abnormalities; ☐Debris (mild / mod / sev) (AU / AD / AS)
☐*Oral cavity*: No abnormalities; ☐Tarter (mild / mod/ sev); ☐Gingivitis
☐*Lymph nodes*: Small, symmetrical, smooth, and soft
☐*Abdomen*: Soft, non-painful, no fluid-wave, organomegaly, or masses
☐*Mammary Chain*: No abnormalities
☐*Penis/ Vulva*: No abnormalities
☐*Skin*: No alopecia, masses, erythema, other lesions, or ectoparasites
☐*Neuro*: No paresis, ataxia, or postural deficits, normal PLR and mentation
☐*MS*: Adequate and symmetrical muscling, no overt lameness
☐*Rectal*: No abnormalities, normal colored feces on glove

Labwork:

Other Diagnostics:
Blood Pressure:

Problem List:

Plan:

Case No._____

Patient		Age	Sex	Breed	Weight
	DOB:		Mn / Mi Fs / Fi	Color:	kg

Owner	Primary Veterinarian	Admit Date/ Time
Name: Phone:	Name: Phone:	Date: Time: AM / PM

• **Presenting Complaint**:_____

_____

_____

• **Medical Hx**:_____

_____

_____

• **When/ where obtained**:   Date:_____; ☐Breeder, ☐Shelter, Other:_____

Drug/ Suppl.	Amount	Dose (mg/kg)	Route	Frequency	Date Started

• **Vaccine status – Dog**: ☐Rab ☐Parv ☐Dist ☐Aden; ☐Para ☐Lep ☐Bord ☐Influ ☐Lyme
• **Vaccine status – Cat**: ☐Rab ☐Herp ☐Cali ☐Pan ☐FeLV[kittens]; ☐FIV ☐Chlam ☐Bord
• **Heartworm / Flea & Tick / Intestinal Parasites**:
  ◦ *Last Heartworm Test*: Date:_____, ☐IDK; Test Results: ☐Pos, ☐Neg, ☐IDK
  ◦ *Monthly heartworm preventative*: ☐no ☐yes, Product:_____
  ◦ *Monthly flea & tick preventative*: ☐no ☐yes, Product:_____
  ◦ *Monthly dewormer*:   ☐no ☐yes, Product:_____
• **Surgical Hx**:   ☐Spay/Neuter; Date:_____; Other:_____
• **Environment**: ☐Indoor, ☐Outdoor, Time spent outdoors/ Other:_____
• **Housemates**: Dogs:_____ Cats:_____ Other:_____
• **Diet**: ☐Wet, ☐Dry; Brand/ Amt.:_____

Appetite	☐Normal, ☐↑, ☐↓
Weight	☐Normal, ☐↑, ☐↓; Past Wt.:_____ kg; Date:_____; Δ:_____
Thirst	☐Normal, ☐↑, ☐↓
Urination	☐Normal, ☐↑, ☐↓, ☐Blood, ☐Strain
Defecation	☐Normal, ☐↑, ☐↓, ☐Blood, ☐Strain, ☐Diarrhea, ☐Mucus
Discharge	☐No, ☐Yes; Onset/ Describe:
Cough/ Sneeze	☐No, ☐Yes; Onset/ Describe:
Vomit	☐No, ☐Yes; Onset/ Describe:
Respiration	☐Normal, ☐↑ Rate, ☐↑ Effort
Energy level	☐Normal, ☐Lethargic, ☐Exercise intolerance

• **Travel Hx**: ☐None, Other:_____
• **Exposure to**: ☐Standing water, ☐Wildlife, ☐Board/daycare, ☐Dog park, ☐Groomer
• **Adverse reactions to food/ meds**: ☐None, Other:_____
• Can give oral meds: ☐no ☐yes; Helpful Tricks:_____

Physical Exam:

T:　　　*P:*　　　*R:*　　　*Wt.:*　　　BCS:　　　*Pain*:　　　*CRT*:

☐*CV*: Regular rhythm, no murmur, normokinetic and synchronous pulses
☐*Resp*: Normal BV sounds/ effort, normal tracheal sounds/ palpation
☐*Attitude*: Bright, alert, and responsive
☐*Hydration/ Perfusion*: MM pink and moist with a CRT of 1-2 sec
☐*Eyes*: No abnormalities
☐*Nose*: No abnormalities
☐*Ears*: No abnormalities;　☐Debris (mild / mod / sev) (AU / AD / AS)
☐*Oral cavity*: No abnormalities;　☐Tarter (mild / mod/ sev);　☐Gingivitis
☐*Lymph nodes*: Small, symmetrical, smooth, and soft
☐*Abdomen*: Soft, non-painful, no fluid-wave, organomegaly, or masses
☐*Mammary Chain*: No abnormalities
☐*Penis/ Vulva*: No abnormalities
☐*Skin*: No alopecia, masses, erythema, other lesions, or ectoparasites
☐*Neuro*: No paresis, ataxia, or postural deficits, normal PLR and mentation
☐*MS*: Adequate and symmetrical muscling, no overt lameness
☐*Rectal*: No abnormalities, normal colored feces on glove

Labwork:

Other Diagnostics:
Blood Pressure:

Problem List:

Plan:

9

Case No._____

Patient	Age	Sex	Breed	Weight
	DOB:	Mn / Mi Fs / Fi	Color:	kg

Owner		Primary Veterinarian	Admit Date/ Time
Name: Phone:		Name: Phone:	Date: Time: AM / PM

• **Presenting Complaint**:_____

_____

_____

• **Medical Hx**:_____

_____

_____

• **When/ where obtained**:   Date:_____ ; ☐Breeder, ☐Shelter, Other:_____

Drug/ Suppl.	Amount	Dose (mg/kg)	Route	Frequency	Date Started

• **Vaccine status – Dog**: ☐Rab ☐Parv ☐Dist ☐Aden; ☐Para ☐Lep ☐Bord ☐Influ ☐Lyme
• **Vaccine status – Cat**: ☐Rab ☐Herp ☐Cali ☐Pan ☐FeLV[kittens]; ☐FIV ☐Chlam ☐Bord
• **Heartworm / Flea & Tick / Intestinal Parasites**:
  ○ *Last Heartworm Test*: Date:_____ , ☐IDK; Test Results: ☐Pos, ☐Neg, ☐IDK
  ○ *Monthly heartworm preventative*:   ☐no ☐yes, Product:_____
  ○ *Monthly flea & tick preventative*:   ☐no ☐yes, Product:_____
  ○ *Monthly dewormer*:   ☐no ☐yes, Product:_____
• **Surgical Hx**: ☐Spay/Neuter; Date:_____ ; Other:_____
• **Environment**: ☐Indoor, ☐Outdoor, Time spent outdoors/ Other:_____
• **Housemates**: Dogs:_____ Cats:_____ Other:_____
• **Diet**: ☐Wet, ☐Dry; Brand/ Amt.:_____

Appetite	☐Normal, ☐↑, ☐↓
Weight	☐Normal, ☐↑, ☐↓; Past Wt.:_____ kg; Date:_____ ; Δ:_____
Thirst	☐Normal, ☐↑, ☐↓
Urination	☐Normal, ☐↑, ☐↓, ☐Blood, ☐Strain
Defecation	☐Normal, ☐↑, ☐↓, ☐Blood, ☐Strain, ☐Diarrhea, ☐Mucus
Discharge	☐No, ☐Yes; Onset/ Describe:
Cough/ Sneeze	☐No, ☐Yes; Onset/ Describe:
Vomit	☐No, ☐Yes; Onset/ Describe:
Respiration	☐Normal, ☐↑ Rate, ☐↑ Effort
Energy level	☐Normal, ☐Lethargic, ☐Exercise intolerance

• **Travel Hx**: ☐None, Other:_____
• **Exposure to**: ☐Standing water, ☐Wildlife, ☐Board/daycare, ☐Dog park, ☐Groomer
• **Adverse reactions to food/ meds**: ☐None, Other:_____
• Can give oral meds: ☐no ☐yes; Helpful Tricks:_____

Physical Exam:

T: P: R: Wt.:   BCS: Pain: CRT:

☐*CV*: Regular rhythm, no murmur, normokinetic and synchronous pulses
☐*Resp*: Normal BV sounds/ effort, normal tracheal sounds/ palpation
☐*Attitude*: Bright, alert, and responsive
☐*Hydration/ Perfusion*: MM pink and moist with a CRT of 1-2 sec
☐*Eyes*: No abnormalities
☐*Nose*: No abnormalities
☐*Ears*: No abnormalities; ☐Debris (mild / mod / sev) (AU / AD / AS)
☐*Oral cavity*: No abnormalities; ☐Tarter (mild / mod/ sev); ☐Gingivitis
☐*Lymph nodes*: Small, symmetrical, smooth, and soft
☐*Abdomen*: Soft, non-painful, no fluid-wave, organomegaly, or masses
☐*Mammary Chain*: No abnormalities
☐*Penis/ Vulva*: No abnormalities
☐*Skin*: No alopecia, masses, erythema, other lesions, or ectoparasites
☐*Neuro*: No paresis, ataxia, or postural deficits, normal PLR and mentation
☐*MS*: Adequate and symmetrical muscling, no overt lameness
☐*Rectal*: No abnormalities, normal colored feces on glove

Labwork:

Other Diagnostics:
Blood Pressure:

Problem List:

Plan:

Case No._____

Patient	Age	Sex		Breed	Weight
	DOB:	Mn / Mi Fs / Fi	Color:		kg

Owner		Primary Veterinarian	Admit Date/ Time
Name: Phone:		Name: Phone:	Date: Time: AM / PM

• **Presenting Complaint**:_____
_____
_____

• **Medical Hx**:_____
_____
_____

• **When/ where obtained**:   Date:_____ ; □Breeder, □Shelter, Other:_____

Drug/ Suppl.	Amount	Dose (mg/kg)	Route	Frequency	Date Started

• **Vaccine status – Dog**: □Rab □Parv □Dist □Aden; □Para □Lep □Bord □Influ □Lyme
• **Vaccine status – Cat**: □Rab □Herp □Cali □Pan □FeLV[kittens]; □FIV □Chlam □Bord
• **Heartworm / Flea & Tick / Intestinal Parasites**:
    ○ *Last Heartworm Test*: Date:_____, □IDK;   Test Results: □Pos, □Neg, □IDK
    ○ *Monthly heartworm preventative*:   □no □yes,   Product:_____
    ○ *Monthly flea & tick preventative*:   □no □yes,   Product:_____
    ○ *Monthly dewormer*:   □no □yes,   Product:_____
• **Surgical Hx**:   □Spay/Neuter; Date:_____ ;   Other:_____
• **Environment**: □Indoor, □Outdoor, Time spent outdoors/ Other:_____
• **Housemates**: Dogs:_____ Cats:_____ Other:_____
• **Diet**: □Wet, □Dry; Brand/ Amt.:_____

Appetite	□Normal, □↑, □↓
Weight	□Normal, □↑, □↓; Past Wt.:_____ kg; Date:_____; Δ:_____
Thirst	□Normal, □↑, □↓
Urination	□Normal, □↑, □↓, □Blood, □Strain
Defecation	□Normal, □↑, □↓, □Blood, □Strain, □Diarrhea, □Mucus
Discharge	□No, □Yes; Onset/ Describe:
Cough/ Sneeze	□No, □Yes; Onset/ Describe:
Vomit	□No, □Yes; Onset/ Describe:
Respiration	□Normal, □↑ Rate, □↑ Effort
Energy level	□Normal, □Lethargic, □Exercise intolerance

• **Travel Hx**: □None, Other:_____
• **Exposure to**: □Standing water, □Wildlife, □Board/daycare, □Dog park, □Groomer
• **Adverse reactions to food/ meds**: □None, Other:_____
• Can give oral meds: □no □yes; Helpful Tricks:_____

Physical Exam:

T: P: R: Wt.:   BCS: Pain: CRT:

☐*CV*: Regular rhythm, no murmur, normokinetic and synchronous pulses
☐*Resp*: Normal BV sounds/ effort, normal tracheal sounds/ palpation
☐*Attitude*: Bright, alert, and responsive
☐*Hydration/ Perfusion*: MM pink and moist with a CRT of 1-2 sec
☐*Eyes*: No abnormalities
☐*Nose*: No abnormalities
☐*Ears*: No abnormalities; ☐Debris (mild / mod / sev) (AU / AD / AS)
☐*Oral cavity*: No abnormalities; ☐Tarter (mild / mod/ sev); ☐Gingivitis
☐*Lymph nodes*: Small, symmetrical, smooth, and soft
☐*Abdomen*: Soft, non-painful, no fluid-wave, organomegaly, or masses
☐*Mammary Chain*: No abnormalities
☐*Penis/ Vulva*: No abnormalities
☐*Skin*: No alopecia, masses, erythema, other lesions, or ectoparasites
☐*Neuro*: No paresis, ataxia, or postural deficits, normal PLR and mentation
☐*MS*: Adequate and symmetrical muscling, no overt lameness
☐*Rectal*: No abnormalities, normal colored feces on glove

Labwork:

Other Diagnostics:
Blood Pressure:

Problem List:

Plan:

Case No._____

Patient	Age	Sex	Breed		Weight
	DOB:	Mn / Mi Fs / Fi	Color:		kg

Owner		Primary Veterinarian	Admit Date/ Time
Name: Phone:		Name: Phone:	Date: Time: AM / PM

• **Presenting Complaint**:_____

_____

• **Medical Hx**:_____

_____

• **When/ where obtained**:   Date:_____ ; □Breeder, □Shelter, Other:_____

Drug/ Suppl.	Amount	Dose (mg/kg)	Route	Frequency	Date Started

• **Vaccine status** – **Dog**: □Rab □Parv □Dist □Aden; □Para □Lep □Bord □Influ □Lyme
• **Vaccine status** – **Cat**: □Rab □Herp □Cali □Pan □FeLV[kittens]; □FIV □Chlam □Bord
• **Heartworm / Flea & Tick / Intestinal Parasites**:
  ◦ *Last Heartworm Test*: Date:_____, □IDK; Test Results: □Pos, □Neg, □IDK
  ◦ *Monthly heartworm preventative*: □no □yes, Product:_____
  ◦ *Monthly flea & tick preventative*: □no □yes, Product:_____
  ◦ *Monthly dewormer*:   □no □yes, Product:_____
• **Surgical Hx**:   □Spay/Neuter; Date:_____; Other:_____
• **Environment**: □Indoor, □Outdoor, Time spent outdoors/ Other:_____
• **Housemates**: Dogs:_____ Cats:_____ Other:_____
• **Diet**: □Wet, □Dry; Brand/ Amt.:_____

Appetite	□Normal, □↑, □↓
Weight	□Normal, □↑, □↓; Past Wt.:_____ kg; Date:_____ ; Δ:_____
Thirst	□Normal, □↑, □↓
Urination	□Normal, □↑, □↓, □Blood, □Strain
Defecation	□Normal, □↑, □↓, □Blood, □Strain, □Diarrhea, □Mucus
Discharge	□No, □Yes; Onset/ Describe:
Cough/ Sneeze	□No, □Yes; Onset/ Describe:
Vomit	□No, □Yes; Onset/ Describe:
Respiration	□Normal, □↑ Rate, □↑ Effort
Energy level	□Normal, □Lethargic, □Exercise intolerance

• **Travel Hx**: □None, Other:_____
• **Exposure to**: □Standing water, □Wildlife, □Board/daycare, □Dog park, □Groomer
• **Adverse reactions to food/ meds**: □None, Other:_____
• Can give oral meds: □no □yes; Helpful Tricks:_____

Physical Exam:

T: *P:*   *R:*   *Wt.:*   BCS: *Pain*:   *CRT*:

☐*CV*: Regular rhythm, no murmur, normokinetic and synchronous pulses
☐*Resp*: Normal BV sounds/ effort, normal tracheal sounds/ palpation
☐*Attitude*: Bright, alert, and responsive
☐*Hydration/ Perfusion*: MM pink and moist with a CRT of 1-2 sec
☐*Eyes*: No abnormalities
☐*Nose*: No abnormalities
☐*Ears*: No abnormalities; ☐Debris (mild / mod / sev) (AU / AD / AS)
☐*Oral cavity*: No abnormalities; ☐Tarter (mild / mod/ sev); ☐Gingivitis
☐*Lymph nodes*: Small, symmetrical, smooth, and soft
☐*Abdomen*: Soft, non-painful, no fluid-wave, organomegaly, or masses
☐*Mammary Chain*: No abnormalities
☐*Penis/ Vulva*: No abnormalities
☐*Skin*: No alopecia, masses, erythema, other lesions, or ectoparasites
☐*Neuro*: No paresis, ataxia, or postural deficits, normal PLR and mentation
☐*MS*: Adequate and symmetrical muscling, no overt lameness
☐*Rectal*: No abnormalities, normal colored feces on glove

Labwork:

Other Diagnostics:
Blood Pressure:

Problem List:

Plan:

Case No._____

Patient	Age	Sex	Breed	Weight
	DOB:	Mn / Mi Fs / Fi	Color:	kg

Owner		Primary Veterinarian	Admit Date/ Time
Name: Phone:		Name: Phone:	Date: Time: AM / PM

• **Presenting Complaint**:_____
_____
_____
_____

• **Medical Hx**:_____
_____
_____

• **When/ where obtained**:   Date:_____; □Breeder, □Shelter, Other:_____

Drug/ Suppl.	Amount	Dose (mg/kg)	Route	Frequency	Date Started

• **Vaccine status – Dog**: □Rab □Parv □Dist □Aden; □Para □Lep □Bord □Influ □Lyme
• **Vaccine status – Cat**: □Rab □Herp □Cali □Pan □FeLV[kittens]; □FIV □Chlam □Bord
• **Heartworm / Flea & Tick / Intestinal Parasites**:
   ◦ *Last Heartworm Test*: Date:_____, □IDK; Test Results: □Pos, □Neg, □IDK
   ◦ *Monthly heartworm preventative*: □no □yes, Product:_____
   ◦ *Monthly flea & tick preventative*: □no □yes, Product:_____
   ◦ *Monthly dewormer*: □no □yes, Product:_____
• **Surgical Hx**: □Spay/Neuter; Date:_____; Other:_____
• **Environment**: □Indoor, □Outdoor, Time spent outdoors/ Other:_____
• **Housemates**: Dogs:_____ Cats:_____ Other:_____
• **Diet**: □Wet, □Dry; Brand/ Amt.:_____

Appetite	□Normal, □↑, □↓
Weight	□Normal, □↑, □↓; Past Wt.:_____ kg; Date:_____; Δ:_____
Thirst	□Normal, □↑, □↓
Urination	□Normal, □↑, □↓, □Blood, □Strain
Defecation	□Normal, □↑, □↓, □Blood, □Strain, □Diarrhea, □Mucus
Discharge	□No, □Yes; Onset/ Describe:
Cough/ Sneeze	□No, □Yes; Onset/ Describe:
Vomit	□No, □Yes; Onset/ Describe:
Respiration	□Normal, □↑ Rate, □↑ Effort
Energy level	□Normal, □Lethargic, □Exercise intolerance

• **Travel Hx**: □None, Other:_____
• **Exposure to**: □Standing water, □Wildlife, □Board/daycare, □Dog park, □Groomer
• **Adverse reactions to food/ meds**: □None, Other:_____
• Can give oral meds: □no □yes; Helpful Tricks:_____

Physical Exam:

T: *P*:   *R*:   *Wt*.:   *BCS*:   *Pain*:   *CRT*:

☐*CV*: Regular rhythm, no murmur, normokinetic and synchronous pulses
☐*Resp*: Normal BV sounds/ effort, normal tracheal sounds/ palpation
☐*Attitude*: Bright, alert, and responsive
☐*Hydration/ Perfusion*: MM pink and moist with a CRT of 1-2 sec
☐*Eyes*: No abnormalities
☐*Nose*: No abnormalities
☐*Ears*: No abnormalities; ☐Debris (mild / mod / sev) (AU / AD / AS)
☐*Oral cavity*: No abnormalities; ☐Tarter (mild / mod/ sev); ☐Gingivitis
☐*Lymph nodes*: Small, symmetrical, smooth, and soft
☐*Abdomen*: Soft, non-painful, no fluid-wave, organomegaly, or masses
☐*Mammary Chain*: No abnormalities
☐*Penis/ Vulva*: No abnormalities
☐*Skin*: No alopecia, masses, erythema, other lesions, or ectoparasites
☐*Neuro*: No paresis, ataxia, or postural deficits, normal PLR and mentation
☐*MS*: Adequate and symmetrical muscling, no overt lameness
☐*Rectal*: No abnormalities, normal colored feces on glove

Labwork:	**Other Diagnostics:**
	Blood Pressure:

Problem List:

Plan:

Case No._____

Patient	Age	Sex	Breed	Weight
	DOB:	Mn / Mi Fs / Fi	Color:	kg

Owner		Primary Veterinarian	Admit Date/ Time
Name: Phone:		Name: Phone:	Date: Time: AM / PM

• **Presenting Complaint**:_____
_____
_____

• **Medical Hx**:_____
_____
_____

• **When/ where obtained**:   Date:_____ ; □Breeder, □Shelter, Other:_____

Drug/ Suppl.	Amount	Dose (mg/kg)	Route	Frequency	Date Started

• **Vaccine status – Dog**: □Rab □Parv □Dist □Aden; □Para □Lep □Bord □Influ □Lyme
• **Vaccine status – Cat**: □Rab □Herp □Cali □Pan □FeLV[kittens]; □FIV □Chlam □Bord
• **Heartworm / Flea & Tick / Intestinal Parasites**:
  ○ *Last Heartworm Test*: Date:_____, □IDK; Test Results: □Pos, □Neg, □IDK
  ○ *Monthly heartworm preventative*: □no □yes, Product:_____
  ○ *Monthly flea & tick preventative*: □no □yes, Product:_____
  ○ *Monthly dewormer*: □no □yes, Product:_____
• **Surgical Hx**: □Spay/Neuter; Date:_____ ; Other:_____
• **Environment**: □Indoor, □Outdoor, Time spent outdoors/ Other:_____
• **Housemates**: Dogs:_____ Cats:_____ Other:_____
• **Diet**: □Wet, □Dry; Brand/ Amt.:_____

Appetite	□Normal, □↑, □↓
Weight	□Normal, □↑, □↓; Past Wt.:_____ kg; Date:_____ ; Δ:_____
Thirst	□Normal, □↑, □↓
Urination	□Normal, □↑, □↓, □Blood, □Strain
Defecation	□Normal, □↑, □↓, □Blood, □Strain, □Diarrhea, □Mucus
Discharge	□No, □Yes; Onset/ Describe:
Cough/ Sneeze	□No, □Yes; Onset/ Describe:
Vomit	□No, □Yes; Onset/ Describe:
Respiration	□Normal, □↑ Rate, □↑ Effort
Energy level	□Normal, □Lethargic, □Exercise intolerance

• **Travel Hx**: □None, Other:_____
• **Exposure to**: □Standing water, □Wildlife, □Board/daycare, □Dog park, □Groomer
• **Adverse reactions to food/ meds**: □None, Other:_____
• Can give oral meds: □no □yes; Helpful Tricks:_____

Physical Exam:

T: P: R: Wt.:   BCS: Pain: CRT:

☐*CV*: Regular rhythm, no murmur, normokinetic and synchronous pulses
☐*Resp*: Normal BV sounds/ effort, normal tracheal sounds/ palpation
☐*Attitude*: Bright, alert, and responsive
☐*Hydration/ Perfusion*: MM pink and moist with a CRT of 1-2 sec
☐*Eyes*: No abnormalities
☐*Nose*: No abnormalities
☐*Ears*: No abnormalities; ☐Debris (mild / mod / sev) (AU / AD / AS)
☐*Oral cavity*: No abnormalities; ☐Tarter (mild / mod/ sev); ☐Gingivitis
☐*Lymph nodes*: Small, symmetrical, smooth, and soft
☐*Abdomen*: Soft, non-painful, no fluid-wave, organomegaly, or masses
☐*Mammary Chain*: No abnormalities
☐*Penis/ Vulva*: No abnormalities
☐*Skin*: No alopecia, masses, erythema, other lesions, or ectoparasites
☐*Neuro*: No paresis, ataxia, or postural deficits, normal PLR and mentation
☐*MS*: Adequate and symmetrical muscling, no overt lameness
☐*Rectal*: No abnormalities, normal colored feces on glove

Labwork:	**Other Diagnostics:**
	Blood Pressure:

Problem List:

Plan:

19

Case No._____

Patient	Age	Sex	Breed	Weight
	DOB:	Mn / Mi Fs / Fi	Color:	kg

Owner		Primary Veterinarian	Admit Date/ Time
Name: Phone:		Name: Phone:	Date: Time:　　　AM / PM

• **Presenting Complaint**: _____
_____
_____

• **Medical Hx**: _____
_____
_____

• **When/ where obtained**:　Date:_____;　□Breeder, □Shelter, Other:_____

Drug/ Suppl.	Amount	Dose (mg/kg)	Route	Frequency	Date Started

• **Vaccine status – Dog**: □Rab □Parv □Dist □Aden; □Para □Lep □Bord □Influ □Lyme
• **Vaccine status – Cat**: □Rab □Herp □Cali □Pan □FeLV[kittens]; □FIV □Chlam □Bord
• **Heartworm / Flea & Tick / Intestinal Parasites**:
   ◦ *Last Heartworm Test*: Date:_____, □IDK;　Test Results: □Pos, □Neg, □IDK
   ◦ *Monthly heartworm preventative*:　□no □yes,　Product:_____
   ◦ *Monthly flea & tick preventative*:　□no □yes,　Product:_____
   ◦ *Monthly dewormer*:　　　　　　　□no □yes,　Product:_____
• **Surgical Hx**:　□Spay/Neuter;　Date:_____;　Other:_____
• **Environment**: □Indoor, □Outdoor, Time spent outdoors/ Other:_____
• **Housemates**: Dogs:_____　Cats:_____　Other:_____
• **Diet**: □Wet, □Dry; Brand/ Amt.:_____

Appetite	□Normal, □↑, □↓
Weight	□Normal, □↑, □↓; Past Wt.:_____ kg; Date:_____; Δ:_____
Thirst	□Normal, □↑, □↓
Urination	□Normal, □↑, □↓, □Blood, □Strain
Defecation	□Normal, □↑, □↓, □Blood, □Strain, □Diarrhea, □Mucus
Discharge	□No, □Yes; Onset/ Describe:
Cough/ Sneeze	□No, □Yes; Onset/ Describe:
Vomit	□No, □Yes; Onset/ Describe:
Respiration	□Normal, □↑ Rate, □↑ Effort
Energy level	□Normal, □Lethargic, □Exercise intolerance

• **Travel Hx**: □None, Other:_____
• **Exposure to**: □Standing water, □Wildlife, □Board/daycare, □Dog park, □Groomer
• **Adverse reactions to food/ meds**: □None, Other:_____
• Can give oral meds: □no □yes; Helpful Tricks:_____

Physical Exam:

T: *P:* *R:* *Wt.:* *BCS:* *Pain:* *CRT:*

☐*CV*: Regular rhythm, no murmur, normokinetic and synchronous pulses
☐*Resp*: Normal BV sounds/ effort, normal tracheal sounds/ palpation
☐*Attitude*: Bright, alert, and responsive
☐*Hydration/ Perfusion*: MM pink and moist with a CRT of 1-2 sec
☐*Eyes*: No abnormalities
☐*Nose*: No abnormalities
☐*Ears*: No abnormalities; ☐Debris (mild / mod / sev) (AU / AD / AS)
☐*Oral cavity*: No abnormalities; ☐Tarter (mild / mod/ sev); ☐Gingivitis
☐*Lymph nodes*: Small, symmetrical, smooth, and soft
☐*Abdomen*: Soft, non-painful, no fluid-wave, organomegaly, or masses
☐*Mammary Chain*: No abnormalities
☐*Penis/ Vulva*: No abnormalities
☐*Skin*: No alopecia, masses, erythema, other lesions, or ectoparasites
☐*Neuro*: No paresis, ataxia, or postural deficits, normal PLR and mentation
☐*MS*: Adequate and symmetrical muscling, no overt lameness
☐*Rectal*: No abnormalities, normal colored feces on glove

Labwork:

Other Diagnostics:
Blood Pressure:

Problem List:

Plan:

21

Patient	Age	Sex	Breed		Weight
	DOB:	Mn / Mi Fs / Fi	Color:		kg

Owner	Primary Veterinarian	Admit Date/ Time
Name: Phone:	Name: Phone:	Date: Time: AM / PM

• **Presenting Complaint**:_____

_____

_____

• **Medical Hx**:_____

_____

_____

• **When/ where obtained**:   Date:_____ ; ☐Breeder, ☐Shelter, Other:_____

Drug/ Suppl.	Amount	Dose (mg/kg)	Route	Frequency	Date Started

• **Vaccine status – Dog**: ☐Rab ☐Parv ☐Dist ☐Aden; ☐Para ☐Lep ☐Bord ☐Influ ☐Lyme
• **Vaccine status – Cat**: ☐Rab ☐Herp ☐Cali ☐Pan ☐FeLV[kittens]; ☐FIV ☐Chlam ☐Bord
• **Heartworm / Flea & Tick / Intestinal Parasites**:
  ◦ *Last Heartworm Test*: Date:_____, ☐IDK; Test Results: ☐Pos, ☐Neg, ☐IDK
  ◦ *Monthly heartworm preventative*:   ☐no ☐yes, Product:_____
  ◦ *Monthly flea & tick preventative*:   ☐no ☐yes, Product:_____
  ◦ *Monthly dewormer*:   ☐no ☐yes, Product:_____
• **Surgical Hx**:   ☐Spay/Neuter; Date:_____ ; Other:_____
• **Environment**: ☐Indoor, ☐Outdoor, Time spent outdoors/ Other:_____
• **Housemates**: Dogs:_____ Cats:_____ Other:_____
• **Diet**: ☐Wet, ☐Dry; Brand/ Amt.:_____

Appetite	☐Normal, ☐↑, ☐↓
Weight	☐Normal, ☐↑, ☐↓; Past Wt.:_____ kg; Date:_____ ; Δ:_____
Thirst	☐Normal, ☐↑, ☐↓
Urination	☐Normal, ☐↑, ☐↓, ☐Blood, ☐Strain
Defecation	☐Normal, ☐↑, ☐↓, ☐Blood, ☐Strain, ☐Diarrhea, ☐Mucus
Discharge	☐No, ☐Yes; Onset/ Describe:
Cough/ Sneeze	☐No, ☐Yes; Onset/ Describe:
Vomit	☐No, ☐Yes; Onset/ Describe:
Respiration	☐Normal, ☐↑ Rate, ☐↑ Effort
Energy level	☐Normal, ☐Lethargic, ☐Exercise intolerance

• **Travel Hx**: ☐None, Other:_____
• **Exposure to**: ☐Standing water, ☐Wildlife, ☐Board/daycare, ☐Dog park, ☐Groomer
• **Adverse reactions to food/ meds**: ☐None, Other:_____
• Can give oral meds: ☐no ☐yes; Helpful Tricks:_____

Physical Exam:

T: *P:*   *R:*   *Wt.:*   BCS: *Pain:*   *CRT:*

☐*CV*: Regular rhythm, no murmur, normokinetic and synchronous pulses
☐*Resp*: Normal BV sounds/ effort, normal tracheal sounds/ palpation
☐*Attitude*: Bright, alert, and responsive
☐*Hydration/ Perfusion*: MM pink and moist with a CRT of 1-2 sec
☐*Eyes*: No abnormalities
☐*Nose*: No abnormalities
☐*Ears*: No abnormalities; ☐Debris (mild / mod / sev) (AU / AD / AS)
☐*Oral cavity*: No abnormalities; ☐Tarter (mild / mod/ sev); ☐Gingivitis
☐*Lymph nodes*: Small, symmetrical, smooth, and soft
☐*Abdomen*: Soft, non-painful, no fluid-wave, organomegaly, or masses
☐*Mammary Chain*: No abnormalities
☐*Penis/ Vulva*: No abnormalities
☐*Skin*: No alopecia, masses, erythema, other lesions, or ectoparasites
☐*Neuro*: No paresis, ataxia, or postural deficits, normal PLR and mentation
☐*MS*: Adequate and symmetrical muscling, no overt lameness
☐*Rectal*: No abnormalities, normal colored feces on glove

Labwork:

Other Diagnostics:
Blood Pressure:

Problem List:

Plan:

Case No._____

Patient	Age	Sex	Breed	Weight
	DOB:	Mn / Mi Fs / Fi	Color:	kg

Owner	Primary Veterinarian	Admit Date/ Time
Name: Phone:	Name: Phone:	Date: Time: AM / PM

• **Presenting Complaint**:_____
_____
_____
_____

• **Medical Hx**:_____
_____
_____
_____

• **When/ where obtained**:   Date:_____; ☐Breeder, ☐Shelter, Other:_____

Drug/ Suppl.	Amount	Dose (mg/kg)	Route	Frequency	Date Started

• **Vaccine status – Dog**: ☐Rab ☐Parv ☐Dist ☐Aden; ☐Para ☐Lep ☐Bord ☐Influ ☐Lyme
• **Vaccine status – Cat**: ☐Rab ☐Herp ☐Cali ☐Pan ☐FeLV[kittens]; ☐FIV ☐Chlam ☐Bord
• **Heartworm / Flea & Tick / Intestinal Parasites**:
  ◦ *Last Heartworm Test*: Date:_____, ☐IDK; Test Results: ☐Pos, ☐Neg, ☐IDK
  ◦ *Monthly heartworm preventative*: ☐no ☐yes, Product:_____
  ◦ *Monthly flea & tick preventative*: ☐no ☐yes, Product:_____
  ◦ *Monthly dewormer*:   ☐no ☐yes, Product:_____
• **Surgical Hx**: ☐Spay/Neuter; Date:_____; Other:_____
• **Environment**: ☐Indoor, ☐Outdoor, Time spent outdoors/ Other:_____
• **Housemates**: Dogs:_____ Cats:_____ Other:_____
• **Diet**: ☐Wet, ☐Dry; Brand/ Amt.:_____

Appetite	☐Normal, ☐↑, ☐↓
Weight	☐Normal, ☐↑, ☐↓; Past Wt.:_____ kg; Date:_____; Δ:_____
Thirst	☐Normal, ☐↑, ☐↓
Urination	☐Normal, ☐↑, ☐↓, ☐Blood, ☐Strain
Defecation	☐Normal, ☐↑, ☐↓, ☐Blood, ☐Strain, ☐Diarrhea, ☐Mucus
Discharge	☐No, ☐Yes; Onset/ Describe:
Cough/ Sneeze	☐No, ☐Yes; Onset/ Describe:
Vomit	☐No, ☐Yes; Onset/ Describe:
Respiration	☐Normal, ☐↑ Rate, ☐↑ Effort
Energy level	☐Normal, ☐Lethargic, ☐Exercise intolerance

• **Travel Hx**: ☐None, Other:_____
• **Exposure to**: ☐Standing water, ☐Wildlife, ☐Board/daycare, ☐Dog park, ☐Groomer
• **Adverse reactions to food/ meds**: ☐None, Other:_____
• Can give oral meds: ☐no ☐yes; Helpful Tricks:_____

Physical Exam:

T: P: R: Wt.:   BCS: Pain: CRT:

☐*CV*: Regular rhythm, no murmur, normokinetic and synchronous pulses
☐*Resp*: Normal BV sounds/ effort, normal tracheal sounds/ palpation
☐*Attitude*: Bright, alert, and responsive
☐*Hydration/ Perfusion*: MM pink and moist with a CRT of 1-2 sec
☐*Eyes*: No abnormalities
☐*Nose*: No abnormalities
☐*Ears*: No abnormalities; ☐Debris (mild / mod / sev) (AU / AD / AS)
☐*Oral cavity*: No abnormalities; ☐Tarter (mild / mod/ sev); ☐Gingivitis
☐*Lymph nodes*: Small, symmetrical, smooth, and soft
☐*Abdomen*: Soft, non-painful, no fluid-wave, organomegaly, or masses
☐*Mammary Chain*: No abnormalities
☐*Penis/ Vulva*: No abnormalities
☐*Skin*: No alopecia, masses, erythema, other lesions, or ectoparasites
☐*Neuro*: No paresis, ataxia, or postural deficits, normal PLR and mentation
☐*MS*: Adequate and symmetrical muscling, no overt lameness
☐*Rectal*: No abnormalities, normal colored feces on glove

Labwork:

Other Diagnostics:
Blood Pressure:

Problem List:

Plan:

Case No._____

Patient	Age	Sex	Breed	Weight
	DOB:	Mn / Mi Fs / Fi	Color:	kg

Owner	Primary Veterinarian	Admit Date/ Time
Name: Phone:	Name: Phone:	Date: Time: AM / PM

• **Presenting Complaint**:_____
_____
_____

• **Medical Hx**:_____
_____
_____

• **When/ where obtained**:   Date:_____ ; □Breeder, □Shelter, Other:_____

Drug/ Suppl.	Amount	Dose (mg/kg)	Route	Frequency	Date Started

• **Vaccine status – Dog**: □Rab □Parv □Dist □Aden; □Para □Lep □Bord □Influ □Lyme
• **Vaccine status – Cat**: □Rab □Herp □Cali □Pan □FeLV[kittens]; □FIV □Chlam □Bord
• **Heartworm / Flea & Tick / Intestinal Parasites**:
  ◦ *Last Heartworm Test*: Date:_____, □IDK;   Test Results: □Pos, □Neg, □IDK
  ◦ *Monthly heartworm preventative*:   □no □yes,   Product:_____
  ◦ *Monthly flea & tick preventative*:   □no □yes,   Product:_____
  ◦ *Monthly dewormer*:   □no □yes,   Product:_____
• **Surgical Hx**:   □Spay/Neuter; Date:_____;   Other:_____
• **Environment**: □Indoor, □Outdoor, Time spent outdoors/ Other:_____
• **Housemates**: Dogs:_____ Cats:_____ Other:_____
• **Diet**: □Wet, □Dry; Brand/ Amt.:_____

Appetite	□Normal, □↑, □↓
Weight	□Normal, □↑, □↓; Past Wt.:_____ kg; Date:_____; Δ:_____
Thirst	□Normal, □↑, □↓
Urination	□Normal, □↑, □↓, □Blood, □Strain
Defecation	□Normal, □↑, □↓, □Blood, □Strain, □Diarrhea, □Mucus
Discharge	□No, □Yes; Onset/ Describe:
Cough/ Sneeze	□No, □Yes; Onset/ Describe:
Vomit	□No, □Yes; Onset/ Describe:
Respiration	□Normal, □↑ Rate, □↑ Effort
Energy level	□Normal, □Lethargic, □Exercise intolerance

• **Travel Hx**: □None, Other:_____
• **Exposure to**: □Standing water, □Wildlife, □Board/daycare, □Dog park, □Groomer
• **Adverse reactions to food/ meds**: □None, Other:_____
• Can give oral meds: □no □yes; Helpful Tricks:_____

Physical Exam:

T: *P:*   *R:*   *Wt.:*   BCS: *Pain:*   *CRT:*

☐*CV*: Regular rhythm, no murmur, normokinetic and synchronous pulses
☐*Resp*: Normal BV sounds/ effort, normal tracheal sounds/ palpation
☐*Attitude*: Bright, alert, and responsive
☐*Hydration/ Perfusion*: MM pink and moist with a CRT of 1-2 sec
☐*Eyes*: No abnormalities
☐*Nose*: No abnormalities
☐*Ears*: No abnormalities; ☐Debris (mild / mod / sev) (AU / AD / AS)
☐*Oral cavity*: No abnormalities; ☐Tarter (mild / mod/ sev); ☐Gingivitis
☐*Lymph nodes*: Small, symmetrical, smooth, and soft
☐*Abdomen*: Soft, non-painful, no fluid-wave, organomegaly, or masses
☐*Mammary Chain*: No abnormalities
☐*Penis/ Vulva*: No abnormalities
☐*Skin*: No alopecia, masses, erythema, other lesions, or ectoparasites
☐*Neuro*: No paresis, ataxia, or postural deficits, normal PLR and mentation
☐*MS*: Adequate and symmetrical muscling, no overt lameness
☐*Rectal*: No abnormalities, normal colored feces on glove

Labwork:

Other Diagnostics:
Blood Pressure:

Problem List:

Plan:

Case No._____

Patient	Age	Sex	Breed	Weight
	DOB:	Mn / Mi Fs / Fi	Color:	kg

Owner	Primary Veterinarian	Admit Date/ Time
Name: Phone:	Name: Phone:	Date: Time: AM / PM

• **Presenting Complaint**:_____
_____
_____
_____

• **Medical Hx**:_____
_____
_____

• **When/ where obtained**:   Date:_____ ; ☐Breeder, ☐Shelter, Other:_____

Drug/ Suppl.	Amount	Dose (mg/kg)	Route	Frequency	Date Started

• **Vaccine status – Dog**: ☐Rab ☐Parv ☐Dist ☐Aden; ☐Para ☐Lep ☐Bord ☐Influ ☐Lyme
• **Vaccine status – Cat**: ☐Rab ☐Herp ☐Cali ☐Pan ☐FeLV[kittens]; ☐FIV ☐Chlam ☐Bord
• **Heartworm / Flea & Tick / Intestinal Parasites**:
  ◦ *Last Heartworm Test*: Date:_____, ☐IDK; Test Results: ☐Pos, ☐Neg, ☐IDK
  ◦ *Monthly heartworm preventative*: ☐no ☐yes, Product:_____
  ◦ *Monthly flea & tick preventative*: ☐no ☐yes, Product:_____
  ◦ *Monthly dewormer*: ☐no ☐yes, Product:_____
• **Surgical Hx**: ☐Spay/Neuter; Date:_____; Other:_____
• **Environment**: ☐Indoor, ☐Outdoor, Time spent outdoors/ Other:_____
• **Housemates**: Dogs:_____ Cats:_____ Other:_____
• **Diet**: ☐Wet, ☐Dry; Brand/ Amt.:_____

Appetite	☐Normal, ☐↑, ☐↓
Weight	☐Normal, ☐↑, ☐↓; Past Wt.:_____ kg; Date:_____; Δ:_____
Thirst	☐Normal, ☐↑, ☐↓
Urination	☐Normal, ☐↑, ☐↓, ☐Blood, ☐Strain
Defecation	☐Normal, ☐↑, ☐↓, ☐Blood, ☐Strain, ☐Diarrhea, ☐Mucus
Discharge	☐No, ☐Yes; Onset/ Describe:
Cough/ Sneeze	☐No, ☐Yes; Onset/ Describe:
Vomit	☐No, ☐Yes; Onset/ Describe:
Respiration	☐Normal, ☐↑ Rate, ☐↑ Effort
Energy level	☐Normal, ☐Lethargic, ☐Exercise intolerance

• **Travel Hx**: ☐None, Other:_____
• **Exposure to**: ☐Standing water, ☐Wildlife, ☐Board/daycare, ☐Dog park, ☐Groomer
• **Adverse reactions to food/ meds**: ☐None, Other:_____
• Can give oral meds: ☐no ☐yes; Helpful Tricks:_____

Physical Exam:

T: *P:*   *R:*   *Wt.:*   *BCS:*   *Pain:*   *CRT:*

☐*CV*: Regular rhythm, no murmur, normokinetic and synchronous pulses
☐*Resp*: Normal BV sounds/ effort, normal tracheal sounds/ palpation
☐*Attitude*: Bright, alert, and responsive
☐*Hydration/ Perfusion*: MM pink and moist with a CRT of 1-2 sec
☐*Eyes*: No abnormalities
☐*Nose*: No abnormalities
☐*Ears*: No abnormalities; ☐Debris (mild / mod / sev) (AU / AD / AS)
☐*Oral cavity*: No abnormalities; ☐Tarter (mild / mod/ sev); ☐Gingivitis
☐*Lymph nodes*: Small, symmetrical, smooth, and soft
☐*Abdomen*: Soft, non-painful, no fluid-wave, organomegaly, or masses
☐*Mammary Chain*: No abnormalities
☐*Penis/ Vulva*: No abnormalities
☐*Skin*: No alopecia, masses, erythema, other lesions, or ectoparasites
☐*Neuro*: No paresis, ataxia, or postural deficits, normal PLR and mentation
☐*MS*: Adequate and symmetrical muscling, no overt lameness
☐*Rectal*: No abnormalities, normal colored feces on glove

Labwork:

Other Diagnostics:
Blood Pressure:

Problem List:

Plan:

Case No._____

Patient	Age	Sex	Breed	Weight
	DOB:	Mn / Mi Fs / Fi	Color:	kg

Owner		Primary Veterinarian	Admit Date/ Time
Name: Phone:		Name: Phone:	Date: Time: AM / PM

• **Presenting Complaint**:_____
_____
_____
_____

• **Medical Hx**:_____
_____
_____

• **When/ where obtained**:   Date:_____; □Breeder, □Shelter, Other:_____

Drug/ Suppl.	Amount	Dose (mg/kg)	Route	Frequency	Date Started

• **Vaccine status – Dog**: □Rab □Parv □Dist □Aden; □Para □Lep □Bord □Influ □Lyme
• **Vaccine status – Cat**: □Rab □Herp □Cali □Pan □FeLV[kittens]; □FIV □Chlam □Bord
• **Heartworm / Flea & Tick / Intestinal Parasites**:
  ◦ *Last Heartworm Test*: Date:_____, □IDK; Test Results: □Pos, □Neg, □IDK
  ◦ *Monthly heartworm preventative*: □no □yes, Product:_____
  ◦ *Monthly flea & tick preventative*: □no □yes, Product:_____
  ◦ *Monthly dewormer*: □no □yes, Product:_____
• **Surgical Hx**:   □Spay/Neuter; Date:_____;   Other:_____
• **Environment**: □Indoor, □Outdoor, Time spent outdoors/ Other:_____
• **Housemates**: Dogs:_____ Cats:_____ Other:_____
• **Diet**: □Wet, □Dry; Brand/ Amt.:_____

Appetite	□Normal, □↑, □↓
Weight	□Normal, □↑, □↓; Past Wt.:_____ kg; Date:_____; Δ:_____
Thirst	□Normal, □↑, □↓
Urination	□Normal, □↑, □↓, □Blood, □Strain
Defecation	□Normal, □↑, □↓, □Blood, □Strain, □Diarrhea, □Mucus
Discharge	□No, □Yes; Onset/ Describe:
Cough/ Sneeze	□No, □Yes; Onset/ Describe:
Vomit	□No, □Yes; Onset/ Describe:
Respiration	□Normal, □↑ Rate, □↑ Effort
Energy level	□Normal, □Lethargic, □Exercise intolerance

• **Travel Hx**: □None, Other:_____
• **Exposure to**: □Standing water, □Wildlife, □Board/daycare, □Dog park, □Groomer
• **Adverse reactions to food/ meds**: □None, Other:_____
• Can give oral meds: □no □yes; Helpful Tricks:_____

Physical Exam:

T: P: R: Wt.:   BCS: Pain: CRT:

☐*CV*: Regular rhythm, no murmur, normokinetic and synchronous pulses
☐*Resp*: Normal BV sounds/ effort, normal tracheal sounds/ palpation
☐*Attitude*: Bright, alert, and responsive
☐*Hydration/ Perfusion*: MM pink and moist with a CRT of 1-2 sec
☐*Eyes*: No abnormalities
☐*Nose*: No abnormalities
☐*Ears*: No abnormalities; ☐Debris (mild / mod / sev) (AU / AD / AS)
☐*Oral cavity*: No abnormalities; ☐Tarter (mild / mod/ sev); ☐Gingivitis
☐*Lymph nodes*: Small, symmetrical, smooth, and soft
☐*Abdomen*: Soft, non-painful, no fluid-wave, organomegaly, or masses
☐*Mammary Chain*: No abnormalities
☐*Penis/ Vulva*: No abnormalities
☐*Skin*: No alopecia, masses, erythema, other lesions, or ectoparasites
☐*Neuro*: No paresis, ataxia, or postural deficits, normal PLR and mentation
☐*MS*: Adequate and symmetrical muscling, no overt lameness
☐*Rectal*: No abnormalities, normal colored feces on glove

Labwork:

Other Diagnostics:
Blood Pressure:

Problem List:

Plan:

31

Case No._____

Patient	Age	Sex	Breed	Weight
	DOB:	Mn / Mi Fs / Fi	Color:	kg

Owner		Primary Veterinarian	Admit Date/ Time
Name: Phone:		Name: Phone:	Date: Time: AM / PM

• **Presenting Complaint**:_____
_____
_____

• **Medical Hx**:_____
_____
_____

• **When/ where obtained**:   Date:_____;   □Breeder, □Shelter, Other:_____

Drug/ Suppl.	Amount	Dose (mg/kg)	Route	Frequency	Date Started

• **Vaccine status – Dog**: □Rab □Parv □Dist □Aden; □Para □Lep □Bord □Influ □Lyme
• **Vaccine status – Cat**: □Rab □Herp □Cali □Pan □FeLV[kittens]; □FIV □Chlam □Bord
• **Heartworm / Flea & Tick / Intestinal Parasites**:
  ◦ *Last Heartworm Test*: Date:_____, □IDK;   Test Results: □Pos, □Neg, □IDK
  ◦ *Monthly heartworm preventative*:   □no □yes,   Product:_____
  ◦ *Monthly flea & tick preventative*:   □no □yes,   Product:_____
  ◦ *Monthly dewormer*:   □no □yes,   Product:_____
• **Surgical Hx**:   □Spay/Neuter;   Date:_____;   Other:_____
• **Environment**: □Indoor, □Outdoor, Time spent outdoors/ Other:_____
• **Housemates**: Dogs:_____ Cats:_____ Other:_____
• **Diet**: □Wet, □Dry; Brand/ Amt.:_____

Appetite	□Normal, □↑, □↓
Weight	□Normal, □↑, □↓; Past Wt.:_____ kg; Date:_____; Δ:_____
Thirst	□Normal, □↑, □↓
Urination	□Normal, □↑, □↓, □Blood, □Strain
Defecation	□Normal, □↑, □↓, □Blood, □Strain, □Diarrhea, □Mucus
Discharge	□No, □Yes; Onset/ Describe:
Cough/ Sneeze	□No, □Yes; Onset/ Describe:
Vomit	□No, □Yes; Onset/ Describe:
Respiration	□Normal, □↑ Rate, □↑ Effort
Energy level	□Normal, □Lethargic, □Exercise intolerance

• **Travel Hx**: □None, Other:_____
• **Exposure to**: □Standing water, □Wildlife, □Board/daycare, □Dog park, □Groomer
• **Adverse reactions to food/ meds**: □None, Other:_____
• Can give oral meds: □no □yes; Helpful Tricks:_____

Physical Exam:

T:　　　*P:*　　　*R:*　　　*Wt.:*　　　BCS:　　　*Pain:*　　　*CRT:*

☐*CV*: Regular rhythm, no murmur, normokinetic and synchronous pulses
☐*Resp*: Normal BV sounds/ effort, normal tracheal sounds/ palpation
☐*Attitude*: Bright, alert, and responsive
☐*Hydration/ Perfusion*: MM pink and moist with a CRT of 1-2 sec
☐*Eyes*: No abnormalities
☐*Nose*: No abnormalities
☐*Ears*: No abnormalities; ☐Debris (mild / mod / sev) (AU / AD / AS)
☐*Oral cavity*: No abnormalities; ☐Tarter (mild / mod/ sev); ☐Gingivitis
☐*Lymph nodes*: Small, symmetrical, smooth, and soft
☐*Abdomen*: Soft, non-painful, no fluid-wave, organomegaly, or masses
☐*Mammary Chain*: No abnormalities
☐*Penis/ Vulva*: No abnormalities
☐*Skin*: No alopecia, masses, erythema, other lesions, or ectoparasites
☐*Neuro*: No paresis, ataxia, or postural deficits, normal PLR and mentation
☐*MS*: Adequate and symmetrical muscling, no overt lameness
☐*Rectal*: No abnormalities, normal colored feces on glove

Labwork:

Other Diagnostics:
Blood Pressure:

Problem List:

Plan:

Patient	Age	Sex	Breed	Weight
	DOB:	Mn / Mi Fs / Fi	Color:	kg

Owner	Primary Veterinarian	Admit Date/ Time
Name: Phone:	Name: Phone:	Date: Time: AM / PM

• **Presenting Complaint**:_____
_____
_____

• **Medical Hx**:_____
_____
_____

• **When/ where obtained**: Date:_____; ☐Breeder, ☐Shelter, Other:_____

Drug/ Suppl.	Amount	Dose (mg/kg)	Route	Frequency	Date Started

• **Vaccine status – Dog**: ☐Rab ☐Parv ☐Dist ☐Aden; ☐Para ☐Lep ☐Bord ☐Influ ☐Lyme
• **Vaccine status – Cat**: ☐Rab ☐Herp ☐Cali ☐Pan ☐FeLV[kittens]; ☐FIV ☐Chlam ☐Bord
• **Heartworm / Flea & Tick / Intestinal Parasites**:
  ◦ *Last Heartworm Test*: Date:_____, ☐IDK; Test Results: ☐Pos, ☐Neg, ☐IDK
  ◦ *Monthly heartworm preventative*: ☐no ☐yes, Product:_____
  ◦ *Monthly flea & tick preventative*: ☐no ☐yes, Product:_____
  ◦ *Monthly dewormer*: ☐no ☐yes, Product:_____
• **Surgical Hx**: ☐Spay/Neuter; Date:_____; Other:_____
• **Environment**: ☐Indoor, ☐Outdoor, Time spent outdoors/ Other:_____
• **Housemates**: Dogs:_____ Cats:_____ Other:_____
• **Diet**: ☐Wet, ☐Dry; Brand/ Amt.:_____

Appetite	☐Normal, ☐↑, ☐↓
Weight	☐Normal, ☐↑, ☐↓; Past Wt.:_____ kg; Date:_____; Δ:_____
Thirst	☐Normal, ☐↑, ☐↓
Urination	☐Normal, ☐↑, ☐↓, ☐Blood, ☐Strain
Defecation	☐Normal, ☐↑, ☐↓, ☐Blood, ☐Strain, ☐Diarrhea, ☐Mucus
Discharge	☐No, ☐Yes; Onset/ Describe:
Cough/ Sneeze	☐No, ☐Yes; Onset/ Describe:
Vomit	☐No, ☐Yes; Onset/ Describe:
Respiration	☐Normal, ☐↑ Rate, ☐↑ Effort
Energy level	☐Normal, ☐Lethargic, ☐Exercise intolerance

• **Travel Hx**: ☐None, Other:_____
• **Exposure to**: ☐Standing water, ☐Wildlife, ☐Board/daycare, ☐Dog park, ☐Groomer
• **Adverse reactions to food/ meds**: ☐None, Other:_____
• Can give oral meds: ☐no ☐yes; Helpful Tricks:_____

Physical Exam:

T: *P:*   *R:*   *Wt.:*   *BCS:*   *Pain:*   *CRT:*

☐*CV*: Regular rhythm, no murmur, normokinetic and synchronous pulses
☐*Resp*: Normal BV sounds/ effort, normal tracheal sounds/ palpation
☐*Attitude*: Bright, alert, and responsive
☐*Hydration/ Perfusion*: MM pink and moist with a CRT of 1-2 sec
☐*Eyes*: No abnormalities
☐*Nose*: No abnormalities
☐*Ears*: No abnormalities; ☐Debris (mild / mod / sev) (AU / AD / AS)
☐*Oral cavity*: No abnormalities; ☐Tarter (mild / mod/ sev); ☐Gingivitis
☐*Lymph nodes*: Small, symmetrical, smooth, and soft
☐*Abdomen*: Soft, non-painful, no fluid-wave, organomegaly, or masses
☐*Mammary Chain*: No abnormalities
☐*Penis/ Vulva*: No abnormalities
☐*Skin*: No alopecia, masses, erythema, other lesions, or ectoparasites
☐*Neuro*: No paresis, ataxia, or postural deficits, normal PLR and mentation
☐*MS*: Adequate and symmetrical muscling, no overt lameness
☐*Rectal*: No abnormalities, normal colored feces on glove

Labwork:

Other Diagnostics:
Blood Pressure:

Problem List:

Plan:

Case No._____

Patient	Age	Sex	Breed		Weight
	DOB:	Mn / Mi Fs / Fi	Color:		kg

Owner		Primary Veterinarian	Admit Date/ Time
Name: Phone:		Name: Phone:	Date: Time: AM / PM

• **Presenting Complaint**:_____
_____
_____

• **Medical Hx**:_____
_____
_____

• **When/ where obtained**:   Date:_____; ☐Breeder, ☐Shelter, Other:_____

Drug/ Suppl.	Amount	Dose (mg/kg)	Route	Frequency	Date Started

• **Vaccine status – Dog**: ☐Rab ☐Parv ☐Dist ☐Aden; ☐Para ☐Lep ☐Bord ☐Influ ☐Lyme
• **Vaccine status – Cat**: ☐Rab ☐Herp ☐Cali ☐Pan ☐FeLV[kittens]; ☐FIV ☐Chlam ☐Bord
• **Heartworm / Flea & Tick / Intestinal Parasites**:
  ◦ *Last Heartworm Test*: Date:_____, ☐IDK; Test Results: ☐Pos, ☐Neg, ☐IDK
  ◦ *Monthly heartworm preventative*: ☐no ☐yes, Product:_____
  ◦ *Monthly flea & tick preventative*: ☐no ☐yes, Product:_____
  ◦ *Monthly dewormer*: ☐no ☐yes, Product:_____
• **Surgical Hx**: ☐Spay/Neuter; Date:_____; Other:_____
• **Environment**: ☐Indoor, ☐Outdoor, Time spent outdoors/ Other:_____
• **Housemates**: Dogs:_____ Cats:_____ Other:_____
• **Diet**: ☐Wet, ☐Dry; Brand/ Amt.:_____

Appetite	☐Normal, ☐↑, ☐↓
Weight	☐Normal, ☐↑, ☐↓; Past Wt.:_____ kg; Date:_____; Δ:_____
Thirst	☐Normal, ☐↑, ☐↓
Urination	☐Normal, ☐↑, ☐↓, ☐Blood, ☐Strain
Defecation	☐Normal, ☐↑, ☐↓, ☐Blood, ☐Strain, ☐Diarrhea, ☐Mucus
Discharge	☐No, ☐Yes; Onset/ Describe:
Cough/ Sneeze	☐No, ☐Yes; Onset/ Describe:
Vomit	☐No, ☐Yes; Onset/ Describe:
Respiration	☐Normal, ☐↑ Rate, ☐↑ Effort
Energy level	☐Normal, ☐Lethargic, ☐Exercise intolerance

• **Travel Hx**: ☐None, Other:_____
• **Exposure to**: ☐Standing water, ☐Wildlife, ☐Board/daycare, ☐Dog park, ☐Groomer
• **Adverse reactions to food/ meds**: ☐None, Other:_____
• Can give oral meds: ☐no ☐yes; Helpful Tricks:_____

Physical Exam:

T: *P*:   *R*:   *Wt.*:   *BCS*:   *Pain*:   *CRT*:

☐*CV*: Regular rhythm, no murmur, normokinetic and synchronous pulses
☐*Resp*: Normal BV sounds/ effort, normal tracheal sounds/ palpation
☐*Attitude*: Bright, alert, and responsive
☐*Hydration/ Perfusion*: MM pink and moist with a CRT of 1-2 sec
☐*Eyes*: No abnormalities
☐*Nose*: No abnormalities
☐*Ears*: No abnormalities; ☐Debris (mild / mod / sev) (AU / AD / AS)
☐*Oral cavity*: No abnormalities; ☐Tarter (mild / mod/ sev); ☐Gingivitis
☐*Lymph nodes*: Small, symmetrical, smooth, and soft
☐*Abdomen*: Soft, non-painful, no fluid-wave, organomegaly, or masses
☐*Mammary Chain*: No abnormalities
☐*Penis/ Vulva*: No abnormalities
☐*Skin*: No alopecia, masses, erythema, other lesions, or ectoparasites
☐*Neuro*: No paresis, ataxia, or postural deficits, normal PLR and mentation
☐*MS*: Adequate and symmetrical muscling, no overt lameness
☐*Rectal*: No abnormalities, normal colored feces on glove

Labwork:

Other Diagnostics:
Blood Pressure:

Problem List:

Plan:

Case No._____

Patient	Age	Sex	Breed	Weight
	DOB:	Mn / Mi Fs / Fi	Color:	kg

Owner	Primary Veterinarian	Admit Date/ Time
Name: Phone:	Name: Phone:	Date: Time: AM / PM

• **Presenting Complaint**:_____
_____
_____

• **Medical Hx**:_____
_____
_____

• **When/ where obtained**:   Date:_____ ; ☐Breeder, ☐Shelter, Other:_____

Drug/ Suppl.	Amount	Dose (mg/kg)	Route	Frequency	Date Started

• **Vaccine status – Dog**: ☐Rab ☐Parv ☐Dist ☐Aden; ☐Para ☐Lep ☐Bord ☐Influ ☐Lyme
• **Vaccine status – Cat**: ☐Rab ☐Herp ☐Cali ☐Pan ☐FeLV[kittens]; ☐FIV ☐Chlam ☐Bord
• **Heartworm / Flea & Tick / Intestinal Parasites**:
  ◦ *Last Heartworm Test*: Date:_____, ☐IDK; Test Results: ☐Pos, ☐Neg, ☐IDK
  ◦ *Monthly heartworm preventative*:   ☐no ☐yes, Product:_____
  ◦ *Monthly flea & tick preventative*:   ☐no ☐yes, Product:_____
  ◦ *Monthly dewormer*:   ☐no ☐yes, Product:_____
• **Surgical Hx**:   ☐Spay/Neuter; Date:_____; Other:_____
• **Environment**: ☐Indoor, ☐Outdoor, Time spent outdoors/ Other:_____
• **Housemates**: Dogs:_____ Cats:_____ Other:_____
• **Diet**: ☐Wet, ☐Dry; Brand/ Amt.:_____

Appetite	☐Normal, ☐↑, ☐↓
Weight	☐Normal, ☐↑, ☐↓; Past Wt.:_____ kg; Date:_____ ; Δ:_____
Thirst	☐Normal, ☐↑, ☐↓
Urination	☐Normal, ☐↑, ☐↓, ☐Blood, ☐Strain
Defecation	☐Normal, ☐↑, ☐↓, ☐Blood, ☐Strain, ☐Diarrhea, ☐Mucus
Discharge	☐No, ☐Yes; Onset/ Describe:
Cough/ Sneeze	☐No, ☐Yes; Onset/ Describe:
Vomit	☐No, ☐Yes; Onset/ Describe:
Respiration	☐Normal, ☐↑ Rate, ☐↑ Effort
Energy level	☐Normal, ☐Lethargic, ☐Exercise intolerance

• **Travel Hx**: ☐None, Other:_____
• **Exposure to**: ☐Standing water, ☐Wildlife, ☐Board/daycare, ☐Dog park, ☐Groomer
• **Adverse reactions to food/ meds**: ☐None, Other:_____
• Can give oral meds: ☐no ☐yes; Helpful Tricks:_____

Physical Exam:

T: P: R: Wt.:   BCS: Pain: CRT:

☐*CV*: Regular rhythm, no murmur, normokinetic and synchronous pulses
☐*Resp*: Normal BV sounds/ effort, normal tracheal sounds/ palpation
☐*Attitude*: Bright, alert, and responsive
☐*Hydration/ Perfusion*: MM pink and moist with a CRT of 1-2 sec
☐*Eyes*: No abnormalities
☐*Nose*: No abnormalities
☐*Ears*: No abnormalities; ☐Debris (mild / mod / sev) (AU / AD / AS)
☐*Oral cavity*: No abnormalities; ☐Tarter (mild / mod/ sev); ☐Gingivitis
☐*Lymph nodes*: Small, symmetrical, smooth, and soft
☐*Abdomen*: Soft, non-painful, no fluid-wave, organomegaly, or masses
☐*Mammary Chain*: No abnormalities
☐*Penis/ Vulva*: No abnormalities
☐*Skin*: No alopecia, masses, erythema, other lesions, or ectoparasites
☐*Neuro*: No paresis, ataxia, or postural deficits, normal PLR and mentation
☐*MS*: Adequate and symmetrical muscling, no overt lameness
☐*Rectal*: No abnormalities, normal colored feces on glove

Labwork:	**Other Diagnostics:**
	Blood Pressure:

Problem List:

Plan:

Case No._____

Patient	Age	Sex	Breed	Weight
	DOB:	Mn / Mi Fs / Fi	Color:	kg

Owner		Primary Veterinarian	Admit Date/ Time
Name: Phone:		Name: Phone:	Date: Time: AM / PM

• **Presenting Complaint**:_____
_____
_____

• **Medical Hx**:_____
_____
_____

• **When/ where obtained**: Date:_____; ☐Breeder, ☐Shelter, Other:_____

Drug/ Suppl.	Amount	Dose (mg/kg)	Route	Frequency	Date Started

• **Vaccine status – Dog**: ☐Rab ☐Parv ☐Dist ☐Aden; ☐Para ☐Lep ☐Bord ☐Influ ☐Lyme
• **Vaccine status – Cat**: ☐Rab ☐Herp ☐Cali ☐Pan ☐FeLV[kittens]; ☐FIV ☐Chlam ☐Bord
• **Heartworm / Flea & Tick / Intestinal Parasites**:
  ◦ *Last Heartworm Test*: Date:_____, ☐IDK; Test Results: ☐Pos, ☐Neg, ☐IDK
  ◦ *Monthly heartworm preventative*: ☐no ☐yes, Product:_____
  ◦ *Monthly flea & tick preventative*: ☐no ☐yes, Product:_____
  ◦ *Monthly dewormer*: ☐no ☐yes, Product:_____
• **Surgical Hx**: ☐Spay/Neuter; Date:_____; Other:_____
• **Environment**: ☐Indoor, ☐Outdoor, Time spent outdoors/ Other:_____
• **Housemates**: Dogs:_____ Cats:_____ Other:_____
• **Diet**: ☐Wet, ☐Dry; Brand/ Amt.:_____

Appetite	☐Normal, ☐↑, ☐↓
Weight	☐Normal, ☐↑, ☐↓; Past Wt.:_____ kg; Date:_____; Δ:_____
Thirst	☐Normal, ☐↑, ☐↓
Urination	☐Normal, ☐↑, ☐↓, ☐Blood, ☐Strain
Defecation	☐Normal, ☐↑, ☐↓, ☐Blood, ☐Strain, ☐Diarrhea, ☐Mucus
Discharge	☐No, ☐Yes; Onset/ Describe:
Cough/ Sneeze	☐No, ☐Yes; Onset/ Describe:
Vomit	☐No, ☐Yes; Onset/ Describe:
Respiration	☐Normal, ☐↑ Rate, ☐↑ Effort
Energy level	☐Normal, ☐Lethargic, ☐Exercise intolerance

• **Travel Hx**: ☐None, Other:_____
• **Exposure to**: ☐Standing water, ☐Wildlife, ☐Board/daycare, ☐Dog park, ☐Groomer
• **Adverse reactions to food/ meds**: ☐None, Other:_____
• Can give oral meds: ☐no ☐yes; Helpful Tricks:_____

Physical Exam:

T: *P:*   *R:*   *Wt.:*   BCS: *Pain:*   *CRT:*

☐*CV*: Regular rhythm, no murmur, normokinetic and synchronous pulses
☐*Resp*: Normal BV sounds/ effort, normal tracheal sounds/ palpation
☐*Attitude*: Bright, alert, and responsive
☐*Hydration/ Perfusion*: MM pink and moist with a CRT of 1-2 sec
☐*Eyes*: No abnormalities
☐*Nose*: No abnormalities
☐*Ears*: No abnormalities; ☐Debris (mild / mod / sev) (AU / AD / AS)
☐*Oral cavity*: No abnormalities; ☐Tarter (mild / mod/ sev); ☐Gingivitis
☐*Lymph nodes*: Small, symmetrical, smooth, and soft
☐*Abdomen*: Soft, non-painful, no fluid-wave, organomegaly, or masses
☐*Mammary Chain*: No abnormalities
☐*Penis/ Vulva*: No abnormalities
☐*Skin*: No alopecia, masses, erythema, other lesions, or ectoparasites
☐*Neuro*: No paresis, ataxia, or postural deficits, normal PLR and mentation
☐*MS*: Adequate and symmetrical muscling, no overt lameness
☐*Rectal*: No abnormalities, normal colored feces on glove

Labwork:

Other Diagnostics:
Blood Pressure:

Problem List:

Plan:

Patient	Age	Sex	Breed	Weight
	DOB:	Mn / Mi Fs / Fi	Color:	kg

Owner	Primary Veterinarian	Admit Date/ Time
Name: Phone:	Name: Phone:	Date: Time: AM / PM

• **Presenting Complaint**:_____
_____
_____

• **Medical Hx**:_____
_____
_____

• **When/ where obtained**:   Date:_____;   □Breeder, □Shelter, Other:_____

Drug/ Suppl.	Amount	Dose (mg/kg)	Route	Frequency	Date Started

• **Vaccine status – Dog**: □Rab □Parv □Dist □Aden; □Para □Lep □Bord □Influ □Lyme
• **Vaccine status – Cat**: □Rab □Herp □Cali □Pan □FeLV[kittens]; □FIV □Chlam □Bord
• **Heartworm / Flea & Tick / Intestinal Parasites**:
  ◦ *Last Heartworm Test*: Date:_____, □IDK; Test Results: □Pos, □Neg, □IDK
  ◦ *Monthly heartworm preventative*:   □no □yes, Product:_____
  ◦ *Monthly flea & tick preventative*:   □no □yes, Product:_____
  ◦ *Monthly dewormer*:   □no □yes, Product:_____
• **Surgical Hx**:   □Spay/Neuter; Date:_____;   Other:_____
• **Environment**: □Indoor, □Outdoor, Time spent outdoors/ Other:_____
• **Housemates**: Dogs:_____ Cats:_____ Other:_____
• **Diet**: □Wet, □Dry; Brand/ Amt.:_____

Appetite	□Normal, □↑, □↓
Weight	□Normal, □↑, □↓; Past Wt.:_____ kg; Date:_____; Δ:_____
Thirst	□Normal, □↑, □↓
Urination	□Normal, □↑, □↓, □Blood, □Strain
Defecation	□Normal, □↑, □↓, □Blood, □Strain, □Diarrhea, □Mucus
Discharge	□No, □Yes; Onset/ Describe:
Cough/ Sneeze	□No, □Yes; Onset/ Describe:
Vomit	□No, □Yes; Onset/ Describe:
Respiration	□Normal, □↑ Rate, □↑ Effort
Energy level	□Normal, □Lethargic, □Exercise intolerance

• **Travel Hx**: □None, Other:_____
• **Exposure to**: □Standing water, □Wildlife, □Board/daycare, □Dog park, □Groomer
• **Adverse reactions to food/ meds**: □None, Other:_____
• Can give oral meds: □no □yes; Helpful Tricks:_____

Physical Exam:

T: P: R: Wt.:   BCS: Pain: CRT:

☐*CV*: Regular rhythm, no murmur, normokinetic and synchronous pulses
☐*Resp*: Normal BV sounds/ effort, normal tracheal sounds/ palpation
☐*Attitude*: Bright, alert, and responsive
☐*Hydration/ Perfusion*: MM pink and moist with a CRT of 1-2 sec
☐*Eyes*: No abnormalities
☐*Nose*: No abnormalities
☐*Ears*: No abnormalities; ☐Debris (mild / mod / sev) (AU / AD / AS)
☐*Oral cavity*: No abnormalities; ☐Tarter (mild / mod/ sev); ☐Gingivitis
☐*Lymph nodes*: Small, symmetrical, smooth, and soft
☐*Abdomen*: Soft, non-painful, no fluid-wave, organomegaly, or masses
☐*Mammary Chain*: No abnormalities
☐*Penis/ Vulva*: No abnormalities
☐*Skin*: No alopecia, masses, erythema, other lesions, or ectoparasites
☐*Neuro*: No paresis, ataxia, or postural deficits, normal PLR and mentation
☐*MS*: Adequate and symmetrical muscling, no overt lameness
☐*Rectal*: No abnormalities, normal colored feces on glove

Labwork:

Other Diagnostics:
Blood Pressure:

Problem List:

Plan:

Case No._____

Patient		Age	Sex	Breed	Weight
	DOB:		Mn / Mi Fs / Fi	Color:	kg

Owner	Primary Veterinarian	Admit Date/ Time
Name: Phone:	Name: Phone:	Date: Time: AM / PM

• **Presenting Complaint**:_____

_____

• **Medical Hx**:_____

_____

• **When/ where obtained**:   Date:_____;   □Breeder, □Shelter, Other:_____

Drug/ Suppl.	Amount	Dose (mg/kg)	Route	Frequency	Date Started

• **Vaccine status – Dog**: □Rab □Parv □Dist □Aden; □Para □Lep □Bord □Influ □Lyme
• **Vaccine status – Cat**: □Rab □Herp □Cali □Pan □FeLV[kittens]; □FIV □Chlam □Bord
• **Heartworm / Flea & Tick / Intestinal Parasites**:
　◦ *Last Heartworm Test*: Date:_____, □IDK; Test Results: □Pos, □Neg, □IDK
　◦ *Monthly heartworm preventative*: □no □yes, Product:_____
　◦ *Monthly flea & tick preventative*: □no □yes, Product:_____
　◦ *Monthly dewormer*:　　　　　　□no □yes, Product:_____
• **Surgical Hx**:   □Spay/Neuter; Date:_____;   Other:_____
• **Environment**: □Indoor, □Outdoor, Time spent outdoors/ Other:_____
• **Housemates**: Dogs:_____ Cats:_____ Other:_____
• **Diet**: □Wet, □Dry; Brand/ Amt.:_____

Appetite	□Normal, □↑, □↓
Weight	□Normal, □↑, □↓; Past Wt.:_____ kg; Date:_____; Δ:_____
Thirst	□Normal, □↑, □↓
Urination	□Normal, □↑, □↓, □Blood, □Strain
Defecation	□Normal, □↑, □↓, □Blood, □Strain, □Diarrhea, □Mucus
Discharge	□No, □Yes; Onset/ Describe:
Cough/ Sneeze	□No, □Yes; Onset/ Describe:
Vomit	□No, □Yes; Onset/ Describe:
Respiration	□Normal, □↑ Rate, □↑ Effort
Energy level	□Normal, □Lethargic, □Exercise intolerance

• **Travel Hx**: □None, Other:_____
• **Exposure to**: □Standing water, □Wildlife, □Board/daycare, □Dog park, □Groomer
• **Adverse reactions to food/ meds**: □None, Other:_____
• Can give oral meds: □no □yes; Helpful Tricks:_____

Physical Exam:

T: *P:*   *R:*   *Wt.:*   BCS: *Pain:*   *CRT:*

☐*CV*: Regular rhythm, no murmur, normokinetic and synchronous pulses
☐*Resp*: Normal BV sounds/ effort, normal tracheal sounds/ palpation
☐*Attitude*: Bright, alert, and responsive
☐*Hydration/ Perfusion*: MM pink and moist with a CRT of 1-2 sec
☐*Eyes*: No abnormalities
☐*Nose*: No abnormalities
☐*Ears*: No abnormalities; ☐Debris (mild / mod / sev) (AU / AD / AS)
☐*Oral cavity*: No abnormalities; ☐Tarter (mild / mod/ sev); ☐Gingivitis
☐*Lymph nodes*: Small, symmetrical, smooth, and soft
☐*Abdomen*: Soft, non-painful, no fluid-wave, organomegaly, or masses
☐*Mammary Chain*: No abnormalities
☐*Penis/ Vulva*: No abnormalities
☐*Skin*: No alopecia, masses, erythema, other lesions, or ectoparasites
☐*Neuro*: No paresis, ataxia, or postural deficits, normal PLR and mentation
☐*MS*: Adequate and symmetrical muscling, no overt lameness
☐*Rectal*: No abnormalities, normal colored feces on glove

Labwork:

Other Diagnostics:
Blood Pressure:

Problem List:

Plan:

Case No._____

Patient	Age	Sex	Breed	Weight
	DOB:	Mn / Mi Fs / Fi	Color:	kg

Owner		Primary Veterinarian	Admit Date/ Time
Name: Phone:		Name: Phone:	Date: Time: AM / PM

• **Presenting Complaint**:_____
_____
_____

• **Medical Hx**:_____
_____
_____

• **When/ where obtained**:   Date:_____; □Breeder, □Shelter, Other:_____

Drug/ Suppl.	Amount	Dose (mg/kg)	Route	Frequency	Date Started

• **Vaccine status** – **Dog**: □Rab □Parv □Dist □Aden; □Para □Lep □Bord □Influ □Lyme
• **Vaccine status** – **Cat**: □Rab □Herp □Cali □Pan □FeLV[kittens]; □FIV □Chlam □Bord
• **Heartworm / Flea & Tick / Intestinal Parasites**:
  ◦ *Last Heartworm Test*: Date:_____, □IDK; Test Results: □Pos, □Neg, □IDK
  ◦ *Monthly heartworm preventative*: □no □yes, Product:_____
  ◦ *Monthly flea & tick preventative*: □no □yes, Product:_____
  ◦ *Monthly dewormer*:   □no □yes, Product:_____
• **Surgical Hx**: □Spay/Neuter; Date:_____; Other:_____
• **Environment**: □Indoor, □Outdoor, Time spent outdoors/ Other:_____
• **Housemates**: Dogs:_____ Cats:_____ Other:_____
• **Diet**: □Wet, □Dry; Brand/ Amt.:_____

Appetite	□Normal, □↑, □↓
Weight	□Normal, □↑, □↓; Past Wt.:_____ kg; Date:_____; Δ:_____
Thirst	□Normal, □↑, □↓
Urination	□Normal, □↑, □↓, □Blood, □Strain
Defecation	□Normal, □↑, □↓, □Blood, □Strain, □Diarrhea, □Mucus
Discharge	□No, □Yes; Onset/ Describe:
Cough/ Sneeze	□No, □Yes; Onset/ Describe:
Vomit	□No, □Yes; Onset/ Describe:
Respiration	□Normal, □↑ Rate, □↑ Effort
Energy level	□Normal, □Lethargic, □Exercise intolerance

• **Travel Hx**: □None, Other:_____
• **Exposure to**: □Standing water, □Wildlife, □Board/daycare, □Dog park, □Groomer
• **Adverse reactions to food/ meds**: □None, Other:_____
• Can give oral meds: □no □yes; Helpful Tricks:_____

Physical Exam:

T: *P:*   *R:*   *Wt.:*   *BCS:*   *Pain:*   *CRT:*

☐*CV*: Regular rhythm, no murmur, normokinetic and synchronous pulses
☐*Resp*: Normal BV sounds/ effort, normal tracheal sounds/ palpation
☐*Attitude*: Bright, alert, and responsive
☐*Hydration/ Perfusion*: MM pink and moist with a CRT of 1-2 sec
☐*Eyes*: No abnormalities
☐*Nose*: No abnormalities
☐*Ears*: No abnormalities; ☐Debris (mild / mod / sev) (AU / AD / AS)
☐*Oral cavity*: No abnormalities; ☐Tarter (mild / mod/ sev); ☐Gingivitis
☐*Lymph nodes*: Small, symmetrical, smooth, and soft
☐*Abdomen*: Soft, non-painful, no fluid-wave, organomegaly, or masses
☐*Mammary Chain*: No abnormalities
☐*Penis/ Vulva*: No abnormalities
☐*Skin*: No alopecia, masses, erythema, other lesions, or ectoparasites
☐*Neuro*: No paresis, ataxia, or postural deficits, normal PLR and mentation
☐*MS*: Adequate and symmetrical muscling, no overt lameness
☐*Rectal*: No abnormalities, normal colored feces on glove

Labwork:

Other Diagnostics:
Blood Pressure:

Problem List:

Plan:

Case No._____

Patient	Age	Sex	Breed	Weight
	DOB:	Mn / Mi Fs / Fi	Color:	kg

Owner	Primary Veterinarian	Admit Date/ Time
Name: Phone:	Name: Phone:	Date: Time: AM / PM

• **Presenting Complaint**:_____

_____

_____

• **Medical Hx**:_____

_____

_____

• **When/ where obtained**:   Date:_____; □Breeder, □Shelter, Other:_____

Drug/ Suppl.	Amount	Dose (mg/kg)	Route	Frequency	Date Started

• **Vaccine status – Dog**: □Rab □Parv □Dist □Aden; □Para □Lep □Bord □Influ □Lyme
• **Vaccine status – Cat**: □Rab □Herp □Cali □Pan □FeLV[kittens]; □FIV □Chlam □Bord
• **Heartworm / Flea & Tick / Intestinal Parasites**:
  ○ *Last Heartworm Test*: Date:_____, □IDK; Test Results: □Pos, □Neg, □IDK
  ○ *Monthly heartworm preventative*: □no □yes, Product:_____
  ○ *Monthly flea & tick preventative*: □no □yes, Product:_____
  ○ *Monthly dewormer*: □no □yes, Product:_____
• **Surgical Hx**: □Spay/Neuter; Date:_____; Other:_____
• **Environment**: □Indoor, □Outdoor, Time spent outdoors/ Other:_____
• **Housemates**: Dogs:_____ Cats:_____ Other:_____
• **Diet**: □Wet, □Dry; Brand/ Amt.:_____

Appetite	□Normal, □↑, □↓
Weight	□Normal, □↑, □↓; Past Wt.:_____ kg; Date:_____; Δ:_____
Thirst	□Normal, □↑, □↓
Urination	□Normal, □↑, □↓, □Blood, □Strain
Defecation	□Normal, □↑, □↓, □Blood, □Strain, □Diarrhea, □Mucus
Discharge	□No, □Yes; Onset/ Describe:
Cough/ Sneeze	□No, □Yes; Onset/ Describe:
Vomit	□No, □Yes; Onset/ Describe:
Respiration	□Normal, □↑ Rate, □↑ Effort
Energy level	□Normal, □Lethargic, □Exercise intolerance

• **Travel Hx**: □None, Other:_____
• **Exposure to**: □Standing water, □Wildlife, □Board/daycare, □Dog park, □Groomer
• **Adverse reactions to food/ meds**: □None, Other:_____
• Can give oral meds: □no □yes; Helpful Tricks:_____

Physical Exam:

T: *P:*   *R:*   *Wt.:*   *BCS:*   *Pain:*   *CRT:*

- ☐*CV*: Regular rhythm, no murmur, normokinetic and synchronous pulses
- ☐*Resp*: Normal BV sounds/ effort, normal tracheal sounds/ palpation
- ☐*Attitude*: Bright, alert, and responsive
- ☐*Hydration/ Perfusion*: MM pink and moist with a CRT of 1-2 sec
- ☐*Eyes*: No abnormalities
- ☐*Nose*: No abnormalities
- ☐*Ears*: No abnormalities; ☐Debris (mild / mod / sev) (AU / AD / AS)
- ☐*Oral cavity*: No abnormalities; ☐Tarter (mild / mod/ sev); ☐Gingivitis
- ☐*Lymph nodes*: Small, symmetrical, smooth, and soft
- ☐*Abdomen*: Soft, non-painful, no fluid-wave, organomegaly, or masses
- ☐*Mammary Chain*: No abnormalities
- ☐*Penis/ Vulva*: No abnormalities
- ☐*Skin*: No alopecia, masses, erythema, other lesions, or ectoparasites
- ☐*Neuro*: No paresis, ataxia, or postural deficits, normal PLR and mentation
- ☐*MS*: Adequate and symmetrical muscling, no overt lameness
- ☐*Rectal*: No abnormalities, normal colored feces on glove

Labwork:

Other Diagnostics:
Blood Pressure:

Problem List:

Plan:

Case No._____

Patient	Age	Sex	Breed	Weight
	DOB:	Mn / Mi Fs / Fi	Color:	kg

Owner	Primary Veterinarian	Admit Date/ Time
Name: Phone:	Name: Phone:	Date: Time: AM / PM

• **Presenting Complaint**: _____
_____
_____

• **Medical Hx**: _____
_____
_____

• **When/ where obtained**:   Date:_____; ☐Breeder, ☐Shelter, Other:_____

Drug/ Suppl.	Amount	Dose (mg/kg)	Route	Frequency	Date Started

• **Vaccine status – Dog**: ☐Rab ☐Parv ☐Dist ☐Aden; ☐Para ☐Lep ☐Bord ☐Influ ☐Lyme
• **Vaccine status – Cat**: ☐Rab ☐Herp ☐Cali ☐Pan ☐FeLV[kittens]; ☐FIV ☐Chlam ☐Bord
• **Heartworm / Flea & Tick / Intestinal Parasites**:
  ◦ *Last Heartworm Test*: Date:_____, ☐IDK; Test Results: ☐Pos, ☐Neg, ☐IDK
  ◦ *Monthly heartworm preventative*: ☐no ☐yes, Product:_____
  ◦ *Monthly flea & tick preventative*: ☐no ☐yes, Product:_____
  ◦ *Monthly dewormer*: ☐no ☐yes, Product:_____
• **Surgical Hx**: ☐Spay/Neuter; Date:_____; Other:_____
• **Environment**: ☐Indoor, ☐Outdoor, Time spent outdoors/ Other:_____
• **Housemates**: Dogs:_____ Cats:_____ Other:_____
• **Diet**: ☐Wet, ☐Dry; Brand/ Amt.:_____

Appetite	☐Normal, ☐↑, ☐↓
Weight	☐Normal, ☐↑, ☐↓; Past Wt.:_____ kg; Date:_____; Δ:_____
Thirst	☐Normal, ☐↑, ☐↓
Urination	☐Normal, ☐↑, ☐↓, ☐Blood, ☐Strain
Defecation	☐Normal, ☐↑, ☐↓, ☐Blood, ☐Strain, ☐Diarrhea, ☐Mucus
Discharge	☐No, ☐Yes; Onset/ Describe:
Cough/ Sneeze	☐No, ☐Yes; Onset/ Describe:
Vomit	☐No, ☐Yes; Onset/ Describe:
Respiration	☐Normal, ☐↑ Rate, ☐↑ Effort
Energy level	☐Normal, ☐Lethargic, ☐Exercise intolerance

• **Travel Hx**: ☐None, Other:_____
• **Exposure to**: ☐Standing water, ☐Wildlife, ☐Board/daycare, ☐Dog park, ☐Groomer
• **Adverse reactions to food/ meds**: ☐None, Other:_____
• Can give oral meds: ☐no ☐yes; Helpful Tricks:_____

Physical Exam:

T: *P:*   *R:*   *Wt.:*   *BCS:*   *Pain:*   *CRT:*

☐*CV*: Regular rhythm, no murmur, normokinetic and synchronous pulses
☐*Resp*: Normal BV sounds/ effort, normal tracheal sounds/ palpation
☐*Attitude*: Bright, alert, and responsive
☐*Hydration/ Perfusion*: MM pink and moist with a CRT of 1-2 sec
☐*Eyes*: No abnormalities
☐*Nose*: No abnormalities
☐*Ears*: No abnormalities; ☐Debris (mild / mod / sev) (AU / AD / AS)
☐*Oral cavity*: No abnormalities; ☐Tarter (mild / mod/ sev); ☐Gingivitis
☐*Lymph nodes*: Small, symmetrical, smooth, and soft
☐*Abdomen*: Soft, non-painful, no fluid-wave, organomegaly, or masses
☐*Mammary Chain*: No abnormalities
☐*Penis/ Vulva*: No abnormalities
☐*Skin*: No alopecia, masses, erythema, other lesions, or ectoparasites
☐*Neuro*: No paresis, ataxia, or postural deficits, normal PLR and mentation
☐*MS*: Adequate and symmetrical muscling, no overt lameness
☐*Rectal*: No abnormalities, normal colored feces on glove

Labwork:

Other Diagnostics:
Blood Pressure:

Problem List:

Plan:

51

Case No._____

Patient		Age	Sex	Breed	Weight
	DOB:		Mn / Mi Fs / Fi	Color:	kg

Owner	Primary Veterinarian	Admit Date/ Time
Name: Phone:	Name: Phone:	Date: Time: AM / PM

• **Presenting Complaint**:_____
_____
_____
_____

• **Medical Hx**:_____
_____
_____

• **When/ where obtained**: Date:_____; ☐Breeder, ☐Shelter, Other:_____

Drug/ Suppl.	Amount	Dose (mg/kg)	Route	Frequency	Date Started

• **Vaccine status – Dog**: ☐Rab ☐Parv ☐Dist ☐Aden; ☐Para ☐Lep ☐Bord ☐Influ ☐Lyme
• **Vaccine status – Cat**: ☐Rab ☐Herp ☐Cali ☐Pan ☐FeLV[kittens]; ☐FIV ☐Chlam ☐Bord
• **Heartworm / Flea & Tick / Intestinal Parasites**:
    ◦ *Last Heartworm Test*: Date:_____, ☐IDK; Test Results: ☐Pos, ☐Neg, ☐IDK
    ◦ *Monthly heartworm preventative*: ☐no ☐yes, Product:_____
    ◦ *Monthly flea & tick preventative*: ☐no ☐yes, Product:_____
    ◦ *Monthly dewormer*: ☐no ☐yes, Product:_____
• **Surgical Hx**: ☐Spay/Neuter; Date:_____; Other:_____
• **Environment**: ☐Indoor, ☐Outdoor, Time spent outdoors/ Other:_____
• **Housemates**: Dogs:_____ Cats:_____ Other:_____
• **Diet**: ☐Wet, ☐Dry; Brand/ Amt.:_____

Appetite	☐Normal, ☐↑, ☐↓
Weight	☐Normal, ☐↑, ☐↓; Past Wt.:_____ kg; Date:_____; Δ:_____
Thirst	☐Normal, ☐↑, ☐↓
Urination	☐Normal, ☐↑, ☐↓, ☐Blood, ☐Strain
Defecation	☐Normal, ☐↑, ☐↓, ☐Blood, ☐Strain, ☐Diarrhea, ☐Mucus
Discharge	☐No, ☐Yes; Onset/ Describe:
Cough/ Sneeze	☐No, ☐Yes; Onset/ Describe:
Vomit	☐No, ☐Yes; Onset/ Describe:
Respiration	☐Normal, ☐↑ Rate, ☐↑ Effort
Energy level	☐Normal, ☐Lethargic, ☐Exercise intolerance

• **Travel Hx**: ☐None, Other:_____
• **Exposure to**: ☐Standing water, ☐Wildlife, ☐Board/daycare, ☐Dog park, ☐Groomer
• **Adverse reactions to food/ meds**: ☐None, Other:_____
• Can give oral meds: ☐no ☐yes; Helpful Tricks:_____

Physical Exam:

T: *P:*   *R:*   *Wt.:*   *BCS:*   *Pain:*   *CRT:*

☐*CV*: Regular rhythm, no murmur, normokinetic and synchronous pulses
☐*Resp*: Normal BV sounds/ effort, normal tracheal sounds/ palpation
☐*Attitude*: Bright, alert, and responsive
☐*Hydration/ Perfusion*: MM pink and moist with a CRT of 1-2 sec
☐*Eyes*: No abnormalities
☐*Nose*: No abnormalities
☐*Ears*: No abnormalities; ☐Debris (mild / mod / sev) (AU / AD / AS)
☐*Oral cavity*: No abnormalities; ☐Tarter (mild / mod/ sev); ☐Gingivitis
☐*Lymph nodes*: Small, symmetrical, smooth, and soft
☐*Abdomen*: Soft, non-painful, no fluid-wave, organomegaly, or masses
☐*Mammary Chain*: No abnormalities
☐*Penis/ Vulva*: No abnormalities
☐*Skin*: No alopecia, masses, erythema, other lesions, or ectoparasites
☐*Neuro*: No paresis, ataxia, or postural deficits, normal PLR and mentation
☐*MS*: Adequate and symmetrical muscling, no overt lameness
☐*Rectal*: No abnormalities, normal colored feces on glove

Labwork:

Other Diagnostics:
Blood Pressure:

Problem List:

Plan:

Case No._____

Patient	Age	Sex	Breed	Weight
	DOB:	Mn / Mi Fs / Fi	Color:	kg

Owner	Primary Veterinarian	Admit Date/ Time
Name: Phone:	Name: Phone:	Date: Time: AM / PM

• **Presenting Complaint**:_____
_____
_____

• **Medical Hx**:_____
_____
_____

• **When/ where obtained**: Date:_____; □Breeder, □Shelter, Other:_____

Drug/ Suppl.	Amount	Dose (mg/kg)	Route	Frequency	Date Started

• **Vaccine status – Dog**: □Rab □Parv □Dist □Aden; □Para □Lep □Bord □Influ □Lyme
• **Vaccine status – Cat**: □Rab □Herp □Cali □Pan □FeLV[kittens]; □FIV □Chlam □Bord
• **Heartworm / Flea & Tick / Intestinal Parasites**:
  ◦ *Last Heartworm Test*: Date:_____, □IDK; Test Results: □Pos, □Neg, □IDK
  ◦ *Monthly heartworm preventative*: □no □yes, Product:_____
  ◦ *Monthly flea & tick preventative*: □no □yes, Product:_____
  ◦ *Monthly dewormer*: □no □yes, Product:_____
• **Surgical Hx**: □Spay/Neuter; Date:_____; Other:_____
• **Environment**: □Indoor, □Outdoor, Time spent outdoors/ Other:_____
• **Housemates**: Dogs:_____ Cats:_____ Other:_____
• **Diet**: □Wet, □Dry; Brand/ Amt.:_____

Appetite	□Normal, □↑, □↓
Weight	□Normal, □↑, □↓; Past Wt.:_____ kg; Date:_____; Δ:_____
Thirst	□Normal, □↑, □↓
Urination	□Normal, □↑, □↓, □Blood, □Strain
Defecation	□Normal, □↑, □↓, □Blood, □Strain, □Diarrhea, □Mucus
Discharge	□No, □Yes; Onset/ Describe:
Cough/ Sneeze	□No, □Yes; Onset/ Describe:
Vomit	□No, □Yes; Onset/ Describe:
Respiration	□Normal, □↑ Rate, □↑ Effort
Energy level	□Normal, □Lethargic, □Exercise intolerance

• **Travel Hx**: □None, Other:_____
• **Exposure to**: □Standing water, □Wildlife, □Board/daycare, □Dog park, □Groomer
• **Adverse reactions to food/ meds**: □None, Other:_____
• Can give oral meds: □no □yes; Helpful Tricks:_____

Physical Exam:

T: P: R: *Wt.:*   *BCS:*   *Pain:*   *CRT:*

☐*CV*: Regular rhythm, no murmur, normokinetic and synchronous pulses
☐*Resp*: Normal BV sounds/ effort, normal tracheal sounds/ palpation
☐*Attitude*: Bright, alert, and responsive
☐*Hydration/ Perfusion*: MM pink and moist with a CRT of 1-2 sec
☐*Eyes*: No abnormalities
☐*Nose*: No abnormalities
☐*Ears*: No abnormalities; ☐Debris (mild / mod / sev) (AU / AD / AS)
☐*Oral cavity*: No abnormalities; ☐Tarter (mild / mod/ sev); ☐Gingivitis
☐*Lymph nodes*: Small, symmetrical, smooth, and soft
☐*Abdomen*: Soft, non-painful, no fluid-wave, organomegaly, or masses
☐*Mammary Chain*: No abnormalities
☐*Penis/ Vulva*: No abnormalities
☐*Skin*: No alopecia, masses, erythema, other lesions, or ectoparasites
☐*Neuro*: No paresis, ataxia, or postural deficits, normal PLR and mentation
☐*MS*: Adequate and symmetrical muscling, no overt lameness
☐*Rectal*: No abnormalities, normal colored feces on glove

Labwork:

Other Diagnostics:
Blood Pressure:

Problem List:

Plan:

Case No._____

Patient	Age	Sex	Breed	Weight
	DOB:	Mn / Mi Fs / Fi	Color:	kg

Owner	Primary Veterinarian	Admit Date/ Time
Name: Phone:	Name: Phone:	Date: Time: AM / PM

• **Presenting Complaint**:_____

_____

_____

• **Medical Hx**:_____

_____

_____

• **When/ where obtained**:   Date:_____ ; ☐Breeder, ☐Shelter, Other:_____

Drug/ Suppl.	Amount	Dose (mg/kg)	Route	Frequency	Date Started

• **Vaccine status – Dog**: ☐Rab ☐Parv ☐Dist ☐Aden; ☐Para ☐Lep ☐Bord ☐Influ ☐Lyme
• **Vaccine status – Cat**: ☐Rab ☐Herp ☐Cali ☐Pan ☐FeLV[kittens]; ☐FIV ☐Chlam ☐Bord
• **Heartworm / Flea & Tick / Intestinal Parasites**:
  ◦ *Last Heartworm Test*: Date:_____, ☐IDK; Test Results: ☐Pos, ☐Neg, ☐IDK
  ◦ *Monthly heartworm preventative*: ☐no ☐yes, Product:_____
  ◦ *Monthly flea & tick preventative*: ☐no ☐yes, Product:_____
  ◦ *Monthly dewormer*:   ☐no ☐yes, Product:_____
• **Surgical Hx**:   ☐Spay/Neuter; Date:_____; Other:_____
• **Environment**: ☐Indoor, ☐Outdoor, Time spent outdoors/ Other:_____
• **Housemates**: Dogs:_____ Cats:_____ Other:_____
• **Diet**: ☐Wet, ☐Dry; Brand/ Amt.:_____

Appetite	☐Normal, ☐↑, ☐↓
Weight	☐Normal, ☐↑, ☐↓; Past Wt.:_____ kg; Date:_____; Δ:_____
Thirst	☐Normal, ☐↑, ☐↓
Urination	☐Normal, ☐↑, ☐↓, ☐Blood, ☐Strain
Defecation	☐Normal, ☐↑, ☐↓, ☐Blood, ☐Strain, ☐Diarrhea, ☐Mucus
Discharge	☐No, ☐Yes; Onset/ Describe:
Cough/ Sneeze	☐No, ☐Yes; Onset/ Describe:
Vomit	☐No, ☐Yes; Onset/ Describe:
Respiration	☐Normal, ☐↑ Rate, ☐↑ Effort
Energy level	☐Normal, ☐Lethargic, ☐Exercise intolerance

• **Travel Hx**: ☐None, Other:_____
• **Exposure to**: ☐Standing water, ☐Wildlife, ☐Board/daycare, ☐Dog park, ☐Groomer
• **Adverse reactions to food/ meds**: ☐None, Other:_____
• Can give oral meds: ☐no ☐yes; Helpful Tricks:_____

Physical Exam:

T: P: R: Wt.:   BCS: Pain: CRT:

☐*CV*: Regular rhythm, no murmur, normokinetic and synchronous pulses
☐*Resp*: Normal BV sounds/ effort, normal tracheal sounds/ palpation
☐*Attitude*: Bright, alert, and responsive
☐*Hydration/ Perfusion*: MM pink and moist with a CRT of 1-2 sec
☐*Eyes*: No abnormalities
☐*Nose*: No abnormalities
☐*Ears*: No abnormalities; ☐Debris (mild / mod / sev) (AU / AD / AS)
☐*Oral cavity*: No abnormalities; ☐Tarter (mild / mod/ sev); ☐Gingivitis
☐*Lymph nodes*: Small, symmetrical, smooth, and soft
☐*Abdomen*: Soft, non-painful, no fluid-wave, organomegaly, or masses
☐*Mammary Chain*: No abnormalities
☐*Penis/ Vulva*: No abnormalities
☐*Skin*: No alopecia, masses, erythema, other lesions, or ectoparasites
☐*Neuro*: No paresis, ataxia, or postural deficits, normal PLR and mentation
☐*MS*: Adequate and symmetrical muscling, no overt lameness
☐*Rectal*: No abnormalities, normal colored feces on glove

Labwork:

Other Diagnostics:
Blood Pressure:

Problem List:

Plan:

Case No._____

Patient		Age	Sex	Breed	Weight
	DOB:		Mn / Mi Fs / Fi	Color:	kg

Owner	Primary Veterinarian	Admit Date/ Time
Name: Phone:	Name: Phone:	Date: Time: AM / PM

• **Presenting Complaint**:_____
_____
_____

• **Medical Hx**:_____
_____
_____

• **When/ where obtained**:   Date:_____; ☐Breeder, ☐Shelter, Other:_____

Drug/ Suppl.	Amount	Dose (mg/kg)	Route	Frequency	Date Started

• **Vaccine status – Dog**: ☐Rab ☐Parv ☐Dist ☐Aden; ☐Para ☐Lep ☐Bord ☐Influ ☐Lyme
• **Vaccine status – Cat**: ☐Rab ☐Herp ☐Cali ☐Pan ☐FeLV[kittens]; ☐FIV ☐Chlam ☐Bord
• **Heartworm / Flea & Tick / Intestinal Parasites**:
    ◦ *Last Heartworm Test*: Date:_____, ☐IDK; Test Results: ☐Pos, ☐Neg, ☐IDK
    ◦ *Monthly heartworm preventative*:   ☐no ☐yes, Product:_____
    ◦ *Monthly flea & tick preventative*:   ☐no ☐yes, Product:_____
    ◦ *Monthly dewormer*:   ☐no ☐yes, Product:_____
• **Surgical Hx**:   ☐Spay/Neuter; Date:_____; Other:_____
• **Environment**: ☐Indoor, ☐Outdoor, Time spent outdoors/ Other:_____
• **Housemates**: Dogs:_____ Cats:_____ Other:_____
• **Diet**: ☐Wet, ☐Dry; Brand/ Amt.:_____

Appetite	☐Normal, ☐↑, ☐↓
Weight	☐Normal, ☐↑, ☐↓; Past Wt.:_____ kg; Date:_____; Δ:_____
Thirst	☐Normal, ☐↑, ☐↓
Urination	☐Normal, ☐↑, ☐↓, ☐Blood, ☐Strain
Defecation	☐Normal, ☐↑, ☐↓, ☐Blood, ☐Strain, ☐Diarrhea, ☐Mucus
Discharge	☐No, ☐Yes; Onset/ Describe:
Cough/ Sneeze	☐No, ☐Yes; Onset/ Describe:
Vomit	☐No, ☐Yes; Onset/ Describe:
Respiration	☐Normal, ☐↑ Rate, ☐↑ Effort
Energy level	☐Normal, ☐Lethargic, ☐Exercise intolerance

• **Travel Hx**: ☐None, Other:_____
• **Exposure to**: ☐Standing water, ☐Wildlife, ☐Board/daycare, ☐Dog park, ☐Groomer
• **Adverse reactions to food/ meds**: ☐None, Other:_____
• Can give oral meds: ☐no ☐yes; Helpful Tricks:_____

Physical Exam:

T: P: R: Wt.:   BCS: Pain: CRT:

☐*CV*: Regular rhythm, no murmur, normokinetic and synchronous pulses
☐*Resp*: Normal BV sounds/ effort, normal tracheal sounds/ palpation
☐*Attitude*: Bright, alert, and responsive
☐*Hydration/ Perfusion*: MM pink and moist with a CRT of 1-2 sec
☐*Eyes*: No abnormalities
☐*Nose*: No abnormalities
☐*Ears*: No abnormalities; ☐Debris (mild / mod / sev) (AU / AD / AS)
☐*Oral cavity*: No abnormalities; ☐Tarter (mild / mod/ sev); ☐Gingivitis
☐*Lymph nodes*: Small, symmetrical, smooth, and soft
☐*Abdomen*: Soft, non-painful, no fluid-wave, organomegaly, or masses
☐*Mammary Chain*: No abnormalities
☐*Penis/ Vulva*: No abnormalities
☐*Skin*: No alopecia, masses, erythema, other lesions, or ectoparasites
☐*Neuro*: No paresis, ataxia, or postural deficits, normal PLR and mentation
☐*MS*: Adequate and symmetrical muscling, no overt lameness
☐*Rectal*: No abnormalities, normal colored feces on glove

Labwork:

Other Diagnostics:
Blood Pressure:

Problem List:

Plan:

Case No._____

Patient	Age	Sex	Breed	Weight
	DOB:	Mn / Mi Fs / Fi	Color:	kg

Owner		Primary Veterinarian	Admit Date/ Time
Name: Phone:		Name: Phone:	Date: Time: AM / PM

• **Presenting Complaint**:_____

_____

_____

• **Medical Hx**:_____

_____

_____

• **When/ where obtained**:   Date:_____; □Breeder, □Shelter, Other:_____

Drug/ Suppl.	Amount	Dose (mg/kg)	Route	Frequency	Date Started

• **Vaccine status – Dog**: □Rab □Parv □Dist □Aden; □Para □Lep □Bord □Influ □Lyme
• **Vaccine status – Cat**: □Rab □Herp □Cali □Pan □FeLV[kittens]; □FIV □Chlam □Bord
• **Heartworm / Flea & Tick / Intestinal Parasites**:
   ◦ *Last Heartworm Test*: Date:_____, □IDK; Test Results: □Pos, □Neg, □IDK
   ◦ *Monthly heartworm preventative*:   □no □yes, Product:_____
   ◦ *Monthly flea & tick preventative*:   □no □yes, Product:_____
   ◦ *Monthly dewormer*:   □no □yes, Product:_____
• **Surgical Hx**:   □Spay/Neuter; Date:_____; Other:_____
• **Environment**: □Indoor, □Outdoor, Time spent outdoors/ Other:_____
• **Housemates**: Dogs:_____ Cats:_____ Other:_____
• **Diet**: □Wet, □Dry; Brand/ Amt.:_____

Appetite	□Normal, □↑, □↓
Weight	□Normal, □↑, □↓; Past Wt.:_____ kg; Date:_____; Δ:_____
Thirst	□Normal, □↑, □↓
Urination	□Normal, □↑, □↓, □Blood, □Strain
Defecation	□Normal, □↑, □↓, □Blood, □Strain, □Diarrhea, □Mucus
Discharge	□No, □Yes; Onset/ Describe:
Cough/ Sneeze	□No, □Yes; Onset/ Describe:
Vomit	□No, □Yes; Onset/ Describe:
Respiration	□Normal, □↑ Rate, □↑ Effort
Energy level	□Normal, □Lethargic, □Exercise intolerance

• **Travel Hx**: □None, Other:_____
• **Exposure to**: □Standing water, □Wildlife, □Board/daycare, □Dog park, □Groomer
• **Adverse reactions to food/ meds**: □None, Other:_____
• Can give oral meds: □no □yes; Helpful Tricks:_____

Physical Exam:

T: *P*:   *R*:   *Wt.*:   *BCS*:   *Pain*:   *CRT*:

☐*CV*: Regular rhythm, no murmur, normokinetic and synchronous pulses
☐*Resp*: Normal BV sounds/ effort, normal tracheal sounds/ palpation
☐*Attitude*: Bright, alert, and responsive
☐*Hydration/ Perfusion*: MM pink and moist with a CRT of 1-2 sec
☐*Eyes*: No abnormalities
☐*Nose*: No abnormalities
☐*Ears*: No abnormalities; ☐Debris (mild / mod / sev) (AU / AD / AS)
☐*Oral cavity*: No abnormalities; ☐Tarter (mild / mod/ sev); ☐Gingivitis
☐*Lymph nodes*: Small, symmetrical, smooth, and soft
☐*Abdomen*: Soft, non-painful, no fluid-wave, organomegaly, or masses
☐*Mammary Chain*: No abnormalities
☐*Penis/ Vulva*: No abnormalities
☐*Skin*: No alopecia, masses, erythema, other lesions, or ectoparasites
☐*Neuro*: No paresis, ataxia, or postural deficits, normal PLR and mentation
☐*MS*: Adequate and symmetrical muscling, no overt lameness
☐*Rectal*: No abnormalities, normal colored feces on glove

Labwork:

Other Diagnostics:
Blood Pressure:

Problem List:

Plan:

61

Case No._____

Patient	Age	Sex	Breed	Weight
	DOB:	Mn / Mi Fs / Fi	Color:	kg

Owner	Primary Veterinarian	Admit Date/ Time
Name: Phone:	Name: Phone:	Date: Time: AM / PM

• **Presenting Complaint**:_____
_____
_____

• **Medical Hx**:_____
_____
_____

• **When/ where obtained**:   Date:_____ ; □Breeder, □Shelter, Other:_____

Drug/ Suppl.	Amount	Dose (mg/kg)	Route	Frequency	Date Started

• **Vaccine status – Dog**: □Rab □Parv □Dist □Aden; □Para □Lep □Bord □Influ □Lyme
• **Vaccine status – Cat**: □Rab □Herp □Cali □Pan □FeLV[kittens]; □FIV □Chlam □Bord
• **Heartworm / Flea & Tick / Intestinal Parasites**:
  ◦ *Last Heartworm Test*: Date:_____, □IDK; Test Results: □Pos, □Neg, □IDK
  ◦ *Monthly heartworm preventative*:   □no □yes, Product:_____
  ◦ *Monthly flea & tick preventative*:   □no □yes, Product:_____
  ◦ *Monthly dewormer*:   □no □yes, Product:_____
• **Surgical Hx**:   □Spay/Neuter; Date:_____; Other:_____
• **Environment**: □Indoor, □Outdoor, Time spent outdoors/ Other:_____
• **Housemates**: Dogs:_____ Cats:_____ Other:_____
• **Diet**: □Wet, □Dry; Brand/ Amt.:_____

Appetite	□Normal, □↑, □↓
Weight	□Normal, □↑, □↓; Past Wt.:_____ kg; Date:_____; Δ:_____
Thirst	□Normal, □↑, □↓
Urination	□Normal, □↑, □↓, □Blood, □Strain
Defecation	□Normal, □↑, □↓, □Blood, □Strain, □Diarrhea, □Mucus
Discharge	□No, □Yes; Onset/ Describe:
Cough/ Sneeze	□No, □Yes; Onset/ Describe:
Vomit	□No, □Yes; Onset/ Describe:
Respiration	□Normal, □↑ Rate, □↑ Effort
Energy level	□Normal, □Lethargic, □Exercise intolerance

• **Travel Hx**: □None, Other:_____
• **Exposure to**: □Standing water, □Wildlife, □Board/daycare, □Dog park, □Groomer
• **Adverse reactions to food/ meds**: □None, Other:_____
• Can give oral meds: □no □yes; Helpful Tricks:_____

Physical Exam:

T: P: R: Wt.:   BCS: Pain: CRT:

☐*CV*: Regular rhythm, no murmur, normokinetic and synchronous pulses
☐*Resp*: Normal BV sounds/ effort, normal tracheal sounds/ palpation
☐*Attitude*: Bright, alert, and responsive
☐*Hydration/ Perfusion*: MM pink and moist with a CRT of 1-2 sec
☐*Eyes*: No abnormalities
☐*Nose*: No abnormalities
☐*Ears*: No abnormalities; ☐Debris (mild / mod / sev) (AU / AD / AS)
☐*Oral cavity*: No abnormalities; ☐Tarter (mild / mod/ sev); ☐Gingivitis
☐*Lymph nodes*: Small, symmetrical, smooth, and soft
☐*Abdomen*: Soft, non-painful, no fluid-wave, organomegaly, or masses
☐*Mammary Chain*: No abnormalities
☐*Penis/ Vulva*: No abnormalities
☐*Skin*: No alopecia, masses, erythema, other lesions, or ectoparasites
☐*Neuro*: No paresis, ataxia, or postural deficits, normal PLR and mentation
☐*MS*: Adequate and symmetrical muscling, no overt lameness
☐*Rectal*: No abnormalities, normal colored feces on glove

Labwork:	**Other Diagnostics:**
	Blood Pressure:

Problem List:

Plan:

Case No._____

Patient	Age	Sex	Breed		Weight
	DOB:	Mn / Mi Fs / Fi	Color:		kg

Owner		Primary Veterinarian	Admit Date/ Time
Name: Phone:		Name: Phone:	Date: Time: AM / PM

- **Presenting Complaint**:_____
_____
_____

- **Medical Hx**:_____ .
_____
_____

- **When/ where obtained**: Date:_____; ☐Breeder, ☐Shelter, Other:_____

Drug/ Suppl.	Amount	Dose (mg/kg)	Route	Frequency	Date Started

- **Vaccine status – Dog**: ☐Rab ☐Parv ☐Dist ☐Aden; ☐Para ☐Lep ☐Bord ☐Influ ☐Lyme
- **Vaccine status – Cat**: ☐Rab ☐Herp ☐Cali ☐Pan ☐FeLV[kittens]; ☐FIV ☐Chlam ☐Bord
- **Heartworm / Flea & Tick / Intestinal Parasites**:
  - *Last Heartworm Test*: Date:_____, ☐IDK; Test Results: ☐Pos, ☐Neg, ☐IDK
  - *Monthly heartworm preventative*: ☐no ☐yes, Product:_____
  - *Monthly flea & tick preventative*: ☐no ☐yes, Product:_____
  - *Monthly dewormer*: ☐no ☐yes, Product:_____
- **Surgical Hx**: ☐Spay/Neuter; Date:_____; Other:_____
- **Environment**: ☐Indoor, ☐Outdoor, Time spent outdoors/ Other:_____
- **Housemates**: Dogs:_____ Cats:_____ Other:_____
- **Diet**: ☐Wet, ☐Dry; Brand/ Amt.:_____

Appetite	☐Normal, ☐↑, ☐↓
Weight	☐Normal, ☐↑, ☐↓; Past Wt.:_____ kg; Date:_____; Δ:_____
Thirst	☐Normal, ☐↑, ☐↓
Urination	☐Normal, ☐↑, ☐↓, ☐Blood, ☐Strain
Defecation	☐Normal, ☐↑, ☐↓, ☐Blood, ☐Strain, ☐Diarrhea, ☐Mucus
Discharge	☐No, ☐Yes; Onset/ Describe:
Cough/ Sneeze	☐No, ☐Yes; Onset/ Describe:
Vomit	☐No, ☐Yes; Onset/ Describe:
Respiration	☐Normal, ☐↑ Rate, ☐↑ Effort
Energy level	☐Normal, ☐Lethargic, ☐Exercise intolerance

- **Travel Hx**: ☐None, Other:_____
- **Exposure to**: ☐Standing water, ☐Wildlife, ☐Board/daycare, ☐Dog park, ☐Groomer
- **Adverse reactions to food/ meds**: ☐None, Other:_____
- Can give oral meds: ☐no ☐yes; Helpful Tricks:_____

Physical Exam:
T: P: R: Wt.:   BCS: Pain: CRT:

- ☐*CV*: Regular rhythm, no murmur, normokinetic and synchronous pulses
- ☐*Resp*: Normal BV sounds/ effort, normal tracheal sounds/ palpation
- ☐*Attitude*: Bright, alert, and responsive
- ☐*Hydration/ Perfusion*: MM pink and moist with a CRT of 1-2 sec
- ☐*Eyes*: No abnormalities
- ☐*Nose*: No abnormalities
- ☐*Ears*: No abnormalities; ☐Debris (mild / mod / sev) (AU / AD / AS)
- ☐*Oral cavity*: No abnormalities; ☐Tarter (mild / mod/ sev); ☐Gingivitis
- ☐*Lymph nodes*: Small, symmetrical, smooth, and soft
- ☐*Abdomen*: Soft, non-painful, no fluid-wave, organomegaly, or masses
- ☐*Mammary Chain*: No abnormalities
- ☐*Penis/ Vulva*: No abnormalities
- ☐*Skin*: No alopecia, masses, erythema, other lesions, or ectoparasites
- ☐*Neuro*: No paresis, ataxia, or postural deficits, normal PLR and mentation
- ☐*MS*: Adequate and symmetrical muscling, no overt lameness
- ☐*Rectal*: No abnormalities, normal colored feces on glove

Labwork:	**Other Diagnostics:**
	Blood Pressure:

Problem List:

Plan:

Patient	Age	Sex	Breed	Weight
	DOB:	Mn / Mi Fs / Fi	Color:	kg

Owner		Primary Veterinarian	Admit Date/ Time
Name: Phone:		Name: Phone:	Date: Time: AM / PM

• **Presenting Complaint**:_____
_____
_____

• **Medical Hx**:_____
_____
_____

• **When/ where obtained**:   Date:_____; ☐Breeder, ☐Shelter, Other:_____

Drug/ Suppl.	Amount	Dose (mg/kg)	Route	Frequency	Date Started

• **Vaccine status – Dog**: ☐Rab ☐Parv ☐Dist ☐Aden; ☐Para ☐Lep ☐Bord ☐Influ ☐Lyme
• **Vaccine status – Cat**: ☐Rab ☐Herp ☐Cali ☐Pan ☐FeLV[kittens]; ☐FIV ☐Chlam ☐Bord
• **Heartworm / Flea & Tick / Intestinal Parasites**:
  ◦ *Last Heartworm Test*: Date:_____, ☐IDK; Test Results: ☐Pos, ☐Neg, ☐IDK
  ◦ *Monthly heartworm preventative*: ☐no ☐yes, Product:_____
  ◦ *Monthly flea & tick preventative*: ☐no ☐yes, Product:_____
  ◦ *Monthly dewormer*:   ☐no ☐yes, Product:_____
• **Surgical Hx**:   ☐Spay/Neuter; Date:_____; Other:_____
• **Environment**: ☐Indoor, ☐Outdoor, Time spent outdoors/ Other:_____
• **Housemates**: Dogs:_____ Cats:_____ Other:_____
• **Diet**: ☐Wet, ☐Dry; Brand/ Amt.:_____

Appetite	☐Normal, ☐↑, ☐↓
Weight	☐Normal, ☐↑, ☐↓; Past Wt.:_____ kg; Date:_____; Δ:_____
Thirst	☐Normal, ☐↑, ☐↓
Urination	☐Normal, ☐↑, ☐↓, ☐Blood, ☐Strain
Defecation	☐Normal, ☐↑, ☐↓, ☐Blood, ☐Strain, ☐Diarrhea, ☐Mucus
Discharge	☐No, ☐Yes; Onset/ Describe:
Cough/ Sneeze	☐No, ☐Yes; Onset/ Describe:
Vomit	☐No, ☐Yes; Onset/ Describe:
Respiration	☐Normal, ☐↑ Rate, ☐↑ Effort
Energy level	☐Normal, ☐Lethargic, ☐Exercise intolerance

• **Travel Hx**: ☐None, Other:_____
• **Exposure to**: ☐Standing water, ☐Wildlife, ☐Board/daycare, ☐Dog park, ☐Groomer
• **Adverse reactions to food/ meds**: ☐None, Other:_____
• Can give oral meds: ☐no ☐yes; Helpful Tricks:_____

Physical Exam:

T: *P*:   *R*:   *Wt.*:   *BCS*:   *Pain*:   *CRT*:

☐*CV*: Regular rhythm, no murmur, normokinetic and synchronous pulses
☐*Resp*: Normal BV sounds/ effort, normal tracheal sounds/ palpation
☐*Attitude*: Bright, alert, and responsive
☐*Hydration/ Perfusion*: MM pink and moist with a CRT of 1-2 sec
☐*Eyes*: No abnormalities
☐*Nose*: No abnormalities
☐*Ears*: No abnormalities; ☐Debris (mild / mod / sev) (AU / AD / AS)
☐*Oral cavity*: No abnormalities; ☐Tarter (mild / mod/ sev); ☐Gingivitis
☐*Lymph nodes*: Small, symmetrical, smooth, and soft
☐*Abdomen*: Soft, non-painful, no fluid-wave, organomegaly, or masses
☐*Mammary Chain*: No abnormalities
☐*Penis/ Vulva*: No abnormalities
☐*Skin*: No alopecia, masses, erythema, other lesions, or ectoparasites
☐*Neuro*: No paresis, ataxia, or postural deficits, normal PLR and mentation
☐*MS*: Adequate and symmetrical muscling, no overt lameness
☐*Rectal*: No abnormalities, normal colored feces on glove

Labwork:	Other Diagnostics:
	Blood Pressure:

Problem List:

Plan:

Patient	Age	Sex	Breed	Weight
	DOB:	Mn / Mi Fs / Fi	Color:	kg

Owner		Primary Veterinarian	Admit Date/ Time
Name: Phone:		Name: Phone:	Date: Time: AM / PM

- **Presenting Complaint**:_____
  _____
  _____

- **Medical Hx**:_____
  _____
  _____

- **When/ where obtained**:   Date:_____ ; □Breeder, □Shelter, Other:_____

Drug/ Suppl.	Amount	Dose (mg/kg)	Route	Frequency	Date Started

- **Vaccine status – Dog**: □Rab □Parv □Dist □Aden; □Para □Lep □Bord □Influ □Lyme
- **Vaccine status – Cat**: □Rab □Herp □Cali □Pan □FeLV[kittens]; □FIV □Chlam □Bord
- **Heartworm / Flea & Tick / Intestinal Parasites**:
  - *Last Heartworm Test*: Date:_____, □IDK; Test Results: □Pos, □Neg, □IDK
  - *Monthly heartworm preventative*: □no □yes, Product:_____
  - *Monthly flea & tick preventative*: □no □yes, Product:_____
  - *Monthly dewormer*: □no □yes, Product:_____
- **Surgical Hx**: □Spay/Neuter; Date:_____ ; Other:_____
- **Environment**: □Indoor, □Outdoor, Time spent outdoors/ Other:_____
- **Housemates**: Dogs:_____ Cats:_____ Other:_____
- **Diet**: □Wet, □Dry; Brand/ Amt.:_____

Appetite	□Normal, □↑, □↓
Weight	□Normal, □↑, □↓; Past Wt.:_____ kg; Date:_____ ; Δ:_____
Thirst	□Normal, □↑, □↓
Urination	□Normal, □↑, □↓, □Blood, □Strain
Defecation	□Normal, □↑, □↓, □Blood, □Strain, □Diarrhea, □Mucus
Discharge	□No, □Yes; Onset/ Describe:
Cough/ Sneeze	□No, □Yes; Onset/ Describe:
Vomit	□No, □Yes; Onset/ Describe:
Respiration	□Normal, □↑ Rate, □↑ Effort
Energy level	□Normal, □Lethargic, □Exercise intolerance

- **Travel Hx**: □None, Other:_____
- **Exposure to**: □Standing water, □Wildlife, □Board/daycare, □Dog park, □Groomer
- **Adverse reactions to food/ meds**: □None, Other:_____
- Can give oral meds: □no □yes; Helpful Tricks:_____

Physical Exam:

T: *P:* *R:* *Wt.:* *BCS:* *Pain:* *CRT:*

☐*CV*: Regular rhythm, no murmur, normokinetic and synchronous pulses
☐*Resp*: Normal BV sounds/ effort, normal tracheal sounds/ palpation
☐*Attitude*: Bright, alert, and responsive
☐*Hydration/ Perfusion*: MM pink and moist with a CRT of 1-2 sec
☐*Eyes*: No abnormalities
☐*Nose*: No abnormalities
☐*Ears*: No abnormalities; ☐Debris (mild / mod / sev) (AU / AD / AS)
☐*Oral cavity*: No abnormalities; ☐Tarter (mild / mod/ sev); ☐Gingivitis
☐*Lymph nodes*: Small, symmetrical, smooth, and soft
☐*Abdomen*: Soft, non-painful, no fluid-wave, organomegaly, or masses
☐*Mammary Chain*: No abnormalities
☐*Penis/ Vulva*: No abnormalities
☐*Skin*: No alopecia, masses, erythema, other lesions, or ectoparasites
☐*Neuro*: No paresis, ataxia, or postural deficits, normal PLR and mentation
☐*MS*: Adequate and symmetrical muscling, no overt lameness
☐*Rectal*: No abnormalities, normal colored feces on glove

Labwork:

Other Diagnostics:
Blood Pressure:

Problem List:

Plan:

69

Case No._____

Patient	Age	Sex	Breed		Weight
	DOB:	Mn / Mi Fs / Fi	Color:		kg

Owner	Primary Veterinarian	Admit Date/ Time
Name: Phone:	Name: Phone:	Date: Time: AM / PM

• **Presenting Complaint**:_____
_____
_____

• **Medical Hx**:_____
_____
_____

• **When/ where obtained**:   Date:_____; □Breeder, □Shelter, Other:_____

Drug/ Suppl.	Amount	Dose (mg/kg)	Route	Frequency	Date Started

• **Vaccine status – Dog**: □Rab □Parv □Dist □Aden; □Para □Lep □Bord □Influ □Lyme
• **Vaccine status – Cat**: □Rab □Herp □Cali □Pan □FeLV[kittens]; □FIV □Chlam □Bord
• **Heartworm / Flea & Tick / Intestinal Parasites**:
  ◦ *Last Heartworm Test*: Date:_____, □IDK; Test Results: □Pos, □Neg, □IDK
  ◦ *Monthly heartworm preventative*: □no □yes, Product:_____
  ◦ *Monthly flea & tick preventative*: □no □yes, Product:_____
  ◦ *Monthly dewormer*:   □no □yes, Product:_____
• **Surgical Hx**:   □Spay/Neuter; Date:_____; Other:_____
• **Environment**: □Indoor, □Outdoor, Time spent outdoors/ Other:_____
• **Housemates**: Dogs:_____ Cats:_____ Other:_____
• **Diet**: □Wet, □Dry; Brand/ Amt.:_____

Appetite	□Normal, □↑, □↓
Weight	□Normal, □↑, □↓; Past Wt.:_____ kg; Date:_____; Δ:_____
Thirst	□Normal, □↑, □↓
Urination	□Normal, □↑, □↓, □Blood, □Strain
Defecation	□Normal, □↑, □↓, □Blood, □Strain, □Diarrhea, □Mucus
Discharge	□No, □Yes; Onset/ Describe:
Cough/ Sneeze	□No, □Yes; Onset/ Describe:
Vomit	□No, □Yes; Onset/ Describe:
Respiration	□Normal, □↑ Rate, □↑ Effort
Energy level	□Normal, □Lethargic, □Exercise intolerance

• **Travel Hx**: □None, Other:_____
• **Exposure to**: □Standing water, □Wildlife, □Board/daycare, □Dog park, □Groomer
• **Adverse reactions to food/ meds**: □None, Other:_____
• **Can give oral meds**: □no □yes; Helpful Tricks:_____

Physical Exam:

T: *P:*   *R:*   *Wt.:*   *BCS:*   *Pain:*   *CRT:*

☐*CV*: Regular rhythm, no murmur, normokinetic and synchronous pulses
☐*Resp*: Normal BV sounds/ effort, normal tracheal sounds/ palpation
☐*Attitude*: Bright, alert, and responsive
☐*Hydration/ Perfusion*: MM pink and moist with a CRT of 1-2 sec
☐*Eyes*: No abnormalities
☐*Nose*: No abnormalities
☐*Ears*: No abnormalities; ☐Debris (mild / mod / sev) (AU / AD / AS)
☐*Oral cavity*: No abnormalities; ☐Tarter (mild / mod/ sev); ☐Gingivitis
☐*Lymph nodes*: Small, symmetrical, smooth, and soft
☐*Abdomen*: Soft, non-painful, no fluid-wave, organomegaly, or masses
☐*Mammary Chain*: No abnormalities
☐*Penis/ Vulva*: No abnormalities
☐*Skin*: No alopecia, masses, erythema, other lesions, or ectoparasites
☐*Neuro*: No paresis, ataxia, or postural deficits, normal PLR and mentation
☐*MS*: Adequate and symmetrical muscling, no overt lameness
☐*Rectal*: No abnormalities, normal colored feces on glove

Labwork:	**Other Diagnostics:**
	Blood Pressure:

Problem List:

Plan:

Case No._____

Patient	Age	Sex	Breed	Weight
	DOB:	Mn / Mi Fs / Fi	Color:	kg

Owner		Primary Veterinarian	Admit Date/ Time
Name: Phone:		Name: Phone:	Date: Time: AM / PM

• **Presenting Complaint**:_____
_____
_____
_____

• **Medical Hx**:_____
_____
_____
_____

• **When/ where obtained**:   Date:_____ ; ☐Breeder, ☐Shelter, Other:_____

Drug/ Suppl.	Amount	Dose (mg/kg)	Route	Frequency	Date Started

• **Vaccine status – Dog**: ☐Rab ☐Parv ☐Dist ☐Aden; ☐Para ☐Lep ☐Bord ☐Influ ☐Lyme
• **Vaccine status – Cat**: ☐Rab ☐Herp ☐Cali ☐Pan ☐FeLV[kittens]; ☐FIV ☐Chlam ☐Bord
• **Heartworm / Flea & Tick / Intestinal Parasites**:
   ◦ *Last Heartworm Test*: Date:_____, ☐IDK;   Test Results: ☐Pos, ☐Neg, ☐IDK
   ◦ *Monthly heartworm preventative*:   ☐no ☐yes,   Product:_____
   ◦ *Monthly flea & tick preventative*:   ☐no ☐yes,   Product:_____
   ◦ *Monthly dewormer*:   ☐no ☐yes,   Product:_____
• **Surgical Hx**: ☐Spay/Neuter; Date:_____;   Other:_____
• **Environment**: ☐Indoor, ☐Outdoor, Time spent outdoors/ Other:_____
• **Housemates**: Dogs:_____ Cats:_____ Other:_____
• **Diet**: ☐Wet, ☐Dry; Brand/ Amt.:_____

Appetite	☐Normal, ☐↑, ☐↓
Weight	☐Normal, ☐↑, ☐↓; Past Wt.:_____ kg; Date:_____; Δ:_____
Thirst	☐Normal, ☐↑, ☐↓
Urination	☐Normal, ☐↑, ☐↓, ☐Blood, ☐Strain
Defecation	☐Normal, ☐↑, ☐↓, ☐Blood, ☐Strain, ☐Diarrhea, ☐Mucus
Discharge	☐No, ☐Yes; Onset/ Describe:
Cough/ Sneeze	☐No, ☐Yes; Onset/ Describe:
Vomit	☐No, ☐Yes; Onset/ Describe:
Respiration	☐Normal, ☐↑ Rate, ☐↑ Effort
Energy level	☐Normal, ☐Lethargic, ☐Exercise intolerance

• **Travel Hx**: ☐None, Other:_____
• **Exposure to**: ☐Standing water, ☐Wildlife, ☐Board/daycare, ☐Dog park, ☐Groomer
• **Adverse reactions to food/ meds**: ☐None, Other:_____
• Can give oral meds: ☐no ☐yes; Helpful Tricks:_____

Physical Exam:

T:	*P:*	*R:*	*Wt.:*	*BCS:*	*Pain:*	*CRT:*

☐*CV*: Regular rhythm, no murmur, normokinetic and synchronous pulses
☐*Resp*: Normal BV sounds/ effort, normal tracheal sounds/ palpation
☐*Attitude*: Bright, alert, and responsive
☐*Hydration/ Perfusion*: MM pink and moist with a CRT of 1-2 sec
☐*Eyes*: No abnormalities
☐*Nose*: No abnormalities
☐*Ears*: No abnormalities;   ☐Debris (mild / mod / sev) (AU / AD / AS)
☐*Oral cavity*: No abnormalities;   ☐Tarter (mild / mod/ sev);   ☐Gingivitis
☐*Lymph nodes*: Small, symmetrical, smooth, and soft
☐*Abdomen*: Soft, non-painful, no fluid-wave, organomegaly, or masses
☐*Mammary Chain*: No abnormalities
☐*Penis/ Vulva*: No abnormalities
☐*Skin*: No alopecia, masses, erythema, other lesions, or ectoparasites
☐*Neuro*: No paresis, ataxia, or postural deficits, normal PLR and mentation
☐*MS*: Adequate and symmetrical muscling, no overt lameness
☐*Rectal*: No abnormalities, normal colored feces on glove

Labwork:

Other Diagnostics:
Blood Pressure:

Problem List:

Plan:

Patient	Age	Sex	Breed	Weight
	DOB:	Mn / Mi Fs / Fi	Color:	kg

Owner	Primary Veterinarian	Admit Date/ Time
Name: Phone:	Name: Phone:	Date: Time:　　AM / PM

• **Presenting Complaint**: _____
_____
_____
_____

• **Medical Hx**: _____
_____
_____

• **When/ where obtained**:　Date:_____;　□Breeder, □Shelter, Other:_____

Drug/ Suppl.	Amount	Dose (mg/kg)	Route	Frequency	Date Started

• **Vaccine status – Dog**: □Rab □Parv □Dist □Aden; □Para □Lep □Bord □Influ □Lyme
• **Vaccine status – Cat**: □Rab □Herp □Cali □Pan □FeLV[kittens]; □FIV □Chlam □Bord
• **Heartworm / Flea & Tick / Intestinal Parasites**:
   ○ *Last Heartworm Test*: Date:_____, □IDK;　Test Results: □Pos, □Neg, □IDK
   ○ *Monthly heartworm preventative*:　□no □yes,　Product:_____
   ○ *Monthly flea & tick preventative*:　□no □yes,　Product:_____
   ○ *Monthly dewormer*:　　　　　　　□no □yes,　Product:_____
• **Surgical Hx**:　□Spay/Neuter; Date:_____;　Other:_____
• **Environment**: □Indoor, □Outdoor, Time spent outdoors/ Other:_____
• **Housemates**: Dogs:_____ Cats:_____　Other:_____
• **Diet**: □Wet, □Dry; Brand/ Amt.:_____

Appetite	□Normal, □↑, □↓
Weight	□Normal, □↑, □↓; Past Wt.:_____ kg; Date:_____; Δ:_____
Thirst	□Normal, □↑, □↓
Urination	□Normal, □↑, □↓, □Blood, □Strain
Defecation	□Normal, □↑, □↓, □Blood, □Strain, □Diarrhea, □Mucus
Discharge	□No, □Yes; Onset/ Describe:
Cough/ Sneeze	□No, □Yes; Onset/ Describe:
Vomit	□No, □Yes; Onset/ Describe:
Respiration	□Normal, □↑ Rate, □↑ Effort
Energy level	□Normal, □Lethargic, □Exercise intolerance

• **Travel Hx**: □None, Other:_____
• **Exposure to**: □Standing water, □Wildlife, □Board/daycare, □Dog park, □Groomer
• **Adverse reactions to food/ meds**: □None, Other:_____
• **Can give oral meds**: □no □yes; Helpful Tricks:_____

Physical Exam:

T: P: R: Wt.:   BCS: Pain: CRT:

☐*CV*: Regular rhythm, no murmur, normokinetic and synchronous pulses
☐*Resp*: Normal BV sounds/ effort, normal tracheal sounds/ palpation
☐*Attitude*: Bright, alert, and responsive
☐*Hydration/ Perfusion*: MM pink and moist with a CRT of 1-2 sec
☐*Eyes*: No abnormalities
☐*Nose*: No abnormalities
☐*Ears*: No abnormalities; ☐Debris (mild / mod / sev) (AU / AD / AS)
☐*Oral cavity*: No abnormalities; ☐Tarter (mild / mod/ sev); ☐Gingivitis
☐*Lymph nodes*: Small, symmetrical, smooth, and soft
☐*Abdomen*: Soft, non-painful, no fluid-wave, organomegaly, or masses
☐*Mammary Chain*: No abnormalities
☐*Penis/ Vulva*: No abnormalities
☐*Skin*: No alopecia, masses, erythema, other lesions, or ectoparasites
☐*Neuro*: No paresis, ataxia, or postural deficits, normal PLR and mentation
☐*MS*: Adequate and symmetrical muscling, no overt lameness
☐*Rectal*: No abnormalities, normal colored feces on glove

Labwork:	**Other Diagnostics:**
	Blood Pressure:

Problem List:

Plan:

Patient	Age	Sex	Breed		Weight
	DOB:	Mn / Mi Fs / Fi	Color:		kg

Owner	Primary Veterinarian	Admit Date/ Time
Name: Phone:	Name: Phone:	Date: Time: AM / PM

• **Presenting Complaint**:_____
_____
_____

• **Medical Hx**:_____
_____
_____

• **When/ where obtained**: Date:_____; □Breeder, □Shelter, Other:_____

Drug/ Suppl.	Amount	Dose (mg/kg)	Route	Frequency	Date Started

• **Vaccine status – Dog**: □Rab □Parv □Dist □Aden; □Para □Lep □Bord □Influ □Lyme
• **Vaccine status – Cat**: □Rab □Herp □Cali □Pan □FeLV[kittens]; □FIV □Chlam □Bord
• **Heartworm / Flea & Tick / Intestinal Parasites**:
  ○ *Last Heartworm Test*: Date:_____, □IDK; Test Results: □Pos, □Neg, □IDK
  ○ *Monthly heartworm preventative*: □no □yes, Product:_____
  ○ *Monthly flea & tick preventative*: □no □yes, Product:_____
  ○ *Monthly dewormer*: □no □yes, Product:_____
• **Surgical Hx**: □Spay/Neuter; Date:_____; Other:_____
• **Environment**: □Indoor, □Outdoor, Time spent outdoors/ Other:_____
• **Housemates**: Dogs:_____ Cats:_____ Other:_____
• **Diet**: □Wet, □Dry; Brand/ Amt.:_____

Appetite	□Normal, □↑, □↓
Weight	□Normal, □↑, □↓; Past Wt.:_____ kg; Date:_____; Δ:_____
Thirst	□Normal, □↑, □↓
Urination	□Normal, □↑, □↓, □Blood, □Strain
Defecation	□Normal, □↑, □↓, □Blood, □Strain, □Diarrhea, □Mucus
Discharge	□No, □Yes; Onset/ Describe:
Cough/ Sneeze	□No, □Yes; Onset/ Describe:
Vomit	□No, □Yes; Onset/ Describe:
Respiration	□Normal, □↑ Rate, □↑ Effort
Energy level	□Normal, □Lethargic, □Exercise intolerance

• **Travel Hx**: □None, Other:_____
• **Exposure to**: □Standing water, □Wildlife, □Board/daycare, □Dog park, □Groomer
• **Adverse reactions to food/ meds**: □None, Other:_____
• Can give oral meds: □no □yes; Helpful Tricks:_____

Physical Exam:

T: *P:*   *R:*   *Wt.:*   *BCS:*   *Pain:*   *CRT:*

☐*CV*: Regular rhythm, no murmur, normokinetic and synchronous pulses
☐*Resp*: Normal BV sounds/ effort, normal tracheal sounds/ palpation
☐*Attitude*: Bright, alert, and responsive
☐*Hydration/ Perfusion*: MM pink and moist with a CRT of 1-2 sec
☐*Eyes*: No abnormalities
☐*Nose*: No abnormalities
☐*Ears*: No abnormalities; ☐Debris (mild / mod / sev) (AU / AD / AS)
☐*Oral cavity*: No abnormalities; ☐Tarter (mild / mod/ sev); ☐Gingivitis
☐*Lymph nodes*: Small, symmetrical, smooth, and soft
☐*Abdomen*: Soft, non-painful, no fluid-wave, organomegaly, or masses
☐*Mammary Chain*: No abnormalities
☐*Penis/ Vulva*: No abnormalities
☐*Skin*: No alopecia, masses, erythema, other lesions, or ectoparasites
☐*Neuro*: No paresis, ataxia, or postural deficits, normal PLR and mentation
☐*MS*: Adequate and symmetrical muscling, no overt lameness
☐*Rectal*: No abnormalities, normal colored feces on glove

Labwork:

Other Diagnostics:
Blood Pressure:

Problem List:

Plan:

Case No._____

Patient	Age	Sex	Breed	Weight
	DOB:	Mn / Mi Fs / Fi	Color:	kg

Owner		Primary Veterinarian	Admit Date/ Time
Name: Phone:		Name: Phone:	Date: Time: AM / PM

• **Presenting Complaint**:_____
_____
_____

• **Medical Hx**:_____
_____
_____

• **When/ where obtained**:   Date:_____; ☐Breeder, ☐Shelter, Other:_____

Drug/ Suppl.	Amount	Dose (mg/kg)	Route	Frequency	Date Started

• **Vaccine status – Dog**: ☐Rab ☐Parv ☐Dist ☐Aden; ☐Para ☐Lep ☐Bord ☐Influ ☐Lyme
• **Vaccine status – Cat**: ☐Rab ☐Herp ☐Cali ☐Pan ☐FeLV[kittens]; ☐FIV ☐Chlam ☐Bord
• **Heartworm / Flea & Tick / Intestinal Parasites**:
  ◦ *Last Heartworm Test*: Date:_____, ☐IDK; Test Results: ☐Pos, ☐Neg, ☐IDK
  ◦ *Monthly heartworm preventative*: ☐no ☐yes, Product:_____
  ◦ *Monthly flea & tick preventative*: ☐no ☐yes, Product:_____
  ◦ *Monthly dewormer*:   ☐no ☐yes, Product:_____
• **Surgical Hx**: ☐Spay/Neuter; Date:_____; Other:_____
• **Environment**: ☐Indoor, ☐Outdoor, Time spent outdoors/ Other:_____
• **Housemates**: Dogs:_____ Cats:_____ Other:_____
• **Diet**: ☐Wet, ☐Dry; Brand/ Amt.:_____

Appetite	☐Normal, ☐↑, ☐↓
Weight	☐Normal, ☐↑, ☐↓; Past Wt.:_____ kg; Date:_____; Δ:_____
Thirst	☐Normal, ☐↑, ☐↓
Urination	☐Normal, ☐↑, ☐↓, ☐Blood, ☐Strain
Defecation	☐Normal, ☐↑, ☐↓, ☐Blood, ☐Strain, ☐Diarrhea, ☐Mucus
Discharge	☐No, ☐Yes; Onset/ Describe:
Cough/ Sneeze	☐No, ☐Yes; Onset/ Describe:
Vomit	☐No, ☐Yes; Onset/ Describe:
Respiration	☐Normal, ☐↑ Rate, ☐↑ Effort
Energy level	☐Normal, ☐Lethargic, ☐Exercise intolerance

• **Travel Hx**: ☐None, Other:_____
• **Exposure to**: ☐Standing water, ☐Wildlife, ☐Board/daycare, ☐Dog park, ☐Groomer
• **Adverse reactions to food/ meds**: ☐None, Other:_____
• Can give oral meds: ☐no ☐yes; Helpful Tricks:_____

Physical Exam:

T: P: R: Wt.:   BCS: Pain: CRT:

☐*CV*: Regular rhythm, no murmur, normokinetic and synchronous pulses
☐*Resp*: Normal BV sounds/ effort, normal tracheal sounds/ palpation
☐*Attitude*: Bright, alert, and responsive
☐*Hydration/ Perfusion*: MM pink and moist with a CRT of 1-2 sec
☐*Eyes*: No abnormalities
☐*Nose*: No abnormalities
☐*Ears*: No abnormalities; ☐Debris (mild / mod / sev) (AU / AD / AS)
☐*Oral cavity*: No abnormalities; ☐Tarter (mild / mod/ sev); ☐Gingivitis
☐*Lymph nodes*: Small, symmetrical, smooth, and soft
☐*Abdomen*: Soft, non-painful, no fluid-wave, organomegaly, or masses
☐*Mammary Chain*: No abnormalities
☐*Penis/ Vulva*: No abnormalities
☐*Skin*: No alopecia, masses, erythema, other lesions, or ectoparasites
☐*Neuro*: No paresis, ataxia, or postural deficits, normal PLR and mentation
☐*MS*: Adequate and symmetrical muscling, no overt lameness
☐*Rectal*: No abnormalities, normal colored feces on glove

Labwork:

Other Diagnostics:
Blood Pressure:

Problem List:

Plan:

Case No._____

Patient	Age	Sex	Breed	Weight
	DOB:	Mn / Mi Fs / Fi	Color:	kg

Owner	Primary Veterinarian	Admit Date/ Time
Name: Phone:	Name: Phone:	Date: Time: AM / PM

• **Presenting Complaint**:_____
_____
_____

• **Medical Hx**:_____
_____
_____

• **When/ where obtained**:   Date:_____ ; □Breeder, □Shelter, Other:_____

Drug/ Suppl.	Amount	Dose (mg/kg)	Route	Frequency	Date Started

• **Vaccine status – Dog**: □Rab □Parv □Dist □Aden; □Para □Lep □Bord □Influ □Lyme
• **Vaccine status – Cat**: □Rab □Herp □Cali □Pan □FeLV[kittens]; □FIV □Chlam □Bord
• **Heartworm / Flea & Tick / Intestinal Parasites**:
  ◦ *Last Heartworm Test*: Date:_____, □IDK; Test Results: □Pos, □Neg, □IDK
  ◦ *Monthly heartworm preventative*:   □no □yes, Product:_____
  ◦ *Monthly flea & tick preventative*:   □no □yes, Product:_____
  ◦ *Monthly dewormer*:   □no □yes, Product:_____
• **Surgical Hx**:   □Spay/Neuter; Date:_____; Other:_____
• **Environment**: □Indoor, □Outdoor, Time spent outdoors/ Other:_____
• **Housemates**: Dogs:_____ Cats:_____ Other:_____
• **Diet**: □Wet, □Dry; Brand/ Amt.:_____

Appetite	□Normal, □↑, □↓
Weight	□Normal, □↑, □↓; Past Wt.:_____ kg; Date:_____; Δ:_____
Thirst	□Normal, □↑, □↓
Urination	□Normal, □↑, □↓, □Blood, □Strain
Defecation	□Normal, □↑, □↓, □Blood, □Strain, □Diarrhea, □Mucus
Discharge	□No, □Yes; Onset/ Describe:
Cough/ Sneeze	□No, □Yes; Onset/ Describe:
Vomit	□No, □Yes; Onset/ Describe:
Respiration	□Normal, □↑ Rate, □↑ Effort
Energy level	□Normal, □Lethargic, □Exercise intolerance

• **Travel Hx**: □None, Other:_____
• **Exposure to**: □Standing water, □Wildlife, □Board/daycare, □Dog park, □Groomer
• **Adverse reactions to food/ meds**: □None, Other:_____
• Can give oral meds: □no □yes; Helpful Tricks:_____

Physical Exam:

T:　　　*P:*　　　*R:*　　　*Wt.:*　　　*BCS:*　　　*Pain:*　　　*CRT:*

☐*CV*: Regular rhythm, no murmur, normokinetic and synchronous pulses
☐*Resp*: Normal BV sounds/ effort, normal tracheal sounds/ palpation
☐*Attitude*: Bright, alert, and responsive
☐*Hydration/ Perfusion*: MM pink and moist with a CRT of 1-2 sec
☐*Eyes*: No abnormalities
☐*Nose*: No abnormalities
☐*Ears*: No abnormalities; ☐Debris (mild / mod / sev) (AU / AD / AS)
☐*Oral cavity*: No abnormalities; ☐Tarter (mild / mod/ sev); ☐Gingivitis
☐*Lymph nodes*: Small, symmetrical, smooth, and soft
☐*Abdomen*: Soft, non-painful, no fluid-wave, organomegaly, or masses
☐*Mammary Chain*: No abnormalities
☐*Penis/ Vulva*: No abnormalities
☐*Skin*: No alopecia, masses, erythema, other lesions, or ectoparasites
☐*Neuro*: No paresis, ataxia, or postural deficits, normal PLR and mentation
☐*MS*: Adequate and symmetrical muscling, no overt lameness
☐*Rectal*: No abnormalities, normal colored feces on glove

Labwork:

Other Diagnostics:
Blood Pressure:

Problem List:

Plan:

Case No._____

Patient	Age	Sex	Breed	Weight
	DOB:	Mn / Mi Fs / Fi	Color:	kg

Owner	Primary Veterinarian	Admit Date/ Time
Name: Phone:	Name: Phone:	Date: Time: AM / PM

• **Presenting Complaint**:_____
_____
_____
_____

• **Medical Hx**:_____
_____
_____

• **When/ where obtained**:   Date:_____; □Breeder, □Shelter, Other:_____

Drug/ Suppl.	Amount	Dose (mg/kg)	Route	Frequency	Date Started

• **Vaccine status – Dog**: □Rab □Parv □Dist □Aden; □Para □Lep □Bord □Influ □Lyme
• **Vaccine status – Cat**: □Rab □Herp □Cali □Pan □FeLV[kittens]; □FIV □Chlam □Bord
• **Heartworm / Flea & Tick / Intestinal Parasites**:
  ◦ *Last Heartworm Test*: Date:_____, □IDK; Test Results: □Pos, □Neg, □IDK
  ◦ *Monthly heartworm preventative*: □no □yes, Product:_____
  ◦ *Monthly flea & tick preventative*: □no □yes, Product:_____
  ◦ *Monthly dewormer*: □no □yes, Product:_____
• **Surgical Hx**: □Spay/Neuter; Date:_____; Other:_____
• **Environment**: □Indoor, □Outdoor, Time spent outdoors/ Other:_____
• **Housemates**: Dogs:_____ Cats:_____ Other:_____
• **Diet**: □Wet, □Dry; Brand/ Amt.:_____

Appetite	□Normal, □↑, □↓
Weight	□Normal, □↑, □↓; Past Wt.:_____ kg; Date:_____; Δ:_____
Thirst	□Normal, □↑, □↓
Urination	□Normal, □↑, □↓, □Blood, □Strain
Defecation	□Normal, □↑, □↓, □Blood, □Strain, □Diarrhea, □Mucus
Discharge	□No, □Yes; Onset/ Describe:
Cough/ Sneeze	□No, □Yes; Onset/ Describe:
Vomit	□No, □Yes; Onset/ Describe:
Respiration	□Normal, □↑ Rate, □↑ Effort
Energy level	□Normal, □Lethargic, □Exercise intolerance

• **Travel Hx**: □None, Other:_____
• **Exposure to**: □Standing water, □Wildlife, □Board/daycare, □Dog park, □Groomer
• **Adverse reactions to food/ meds**: □None, Other:_____
• Can give oral meds: □no □yes; Helpful Tricks:_____

Physical Exam:

T: P: R: Wt.:   BCS: Pain: CRT:

☐*CV*: Regular rhythm, no murmur, normokinetic and synchronous pulses
☐*Resp*: Normal BV sounds/ effort, normal tracheal sounds/ palpation
☐*Attitude*: Bright, alert, and responsive
☐*Hydration/ Perfusion*: MM pink and moist with a CRT of 1-2 sec
☐*Eyes*: No abnormalities
☐*Nose*: No abnormalities
☐*Ears*: No abnormalities; ☐Debris (mild / mod / sev) (AU / AD / AS)
☐*Oral cavity*: No abnormalities; ☐Tarter (mild / mod/ sev); ☐Gingivitis
☐*Lymph nodes*: Small, symmetrical, smooth, and soft
☐*Abdomen*: Soft, non-painful, no fluid-wave, organomegaly, or masses
☐*Mammary Chain*: No abnormalities
☐*Penis/ Vulva*: No abnormalities
☐*Skin*: No alopecia, masses, erythema, other lesions, or ectoparasites
☐*Neuro*: No paresis, ataxia, or postural deficits, normal PLR and mentation
☐*MS*: Adequate and symmetrical muscling, no overt lameness
☐*Rectal*: No abnormalities, normal colored feces on glove

Labwork:

Other Diagnostics:
Blood Pressure:

Problem List:

Plan:

Patient	Age	Sex	Breed	Weight
	DOB:	Mn / Mi Fs / Fi	Color:	kg

Owner	Primary Veterinarian	Admit Date/ Time
Name: Phone:	Name: Phone:	Date: Time: AM / PM

- **Presenting Complaint**:_____
  _____
  _____
  _____

- **Medical Hx**:_____
  _____
  _____

- **When/ where obtained**: Date:_____; □Breeder, □Shelter, Other:_____

Drug/ Suppl.	Amount	Dose (mg/kg)	Route	Frequency	Date Started

- **Vaccine status – Dog**: □Rab □Parv □Dist □Aden; □Para □Lep □Bord □Influ □Lyme
- **Vaccine status – Cat**: □Rab □Herp □Cali □Pan □FeLV[kittens]; □FIV □Chlam □Bord
- **Heartworm / Flea & Tick / Intestinal Parasites**:
  - *Last Heartworm Test*: Date:_____, □IDK; Test Results: □Pos, □Neg, □IDK
  - *Monthly heartworm preventative*: □no □yes, Product:_____
  - *Monthly flea & tick preventative*: □no □yes, Product:_____
  - *Monthly dewormer*: □no □yes, Product:_____
- **Surgical Hx**: □Spay/Neuter; Date:_____; Other:_____
- **Environment**: □Indoor, □Outdoor, Time spent outdoors/ Other:_____
- **Housemates**: Dogs:_____ Cats:_____ Other:_____
- **Diet**: □Wet, □Dry; Brand/ Amt.:_____

Appetite	□Normal, □↑, □↓
Weight	□Normal, □↑, □↓; Past Wt.:_____ kg; Date:_____; Δ:_____
Thirst	□Normal, □↑, □↓
Urination	□Normal, □↑, □↓, □Blood, □Strain
Defecation	□Normal, □↑, □↓, □Blood, □Strain, □Diarrhea, □Mucus
Discharge	□No, □Yes; Onset/ Describe:
Cough/ Sneeze	□No, □Yes; Onset/ Describe:
Vomit	□No, □Yes; Onset/ Describe:
Respiration	□Normal, □↑ Rate, □↑ Effort
Energy level	□Normal, □Lethargic, □Exercise intolerance

- **Travel Hx**: □None, Other:_____
- **Exposure to**: □Standing water, □Wildlife, □Board/daycare, □Dog park, □Groomer
- **Adverse reactions to food/ meds**: □None, Other:_____
- Can give oral meds: □no □yes; Helpful Tricks:_____

Physical Exam:

T: P: R: Wt.:   BCS: Pain: CRT:

☐*CV*: Regular rhythm, no murmur, normokinetic and synchronous pulses
☐*Resp*: Normal BV sounds/ effort, normal tracheal sounds/ palpation
☐*Attitude*: Bright, alert, and responsive
☐*Hydration/ Perfusion*: MM pink and moist with a CRT of 1-2 sec
☐*Eyes*: No abnormalities
☐*Nose*: No abnormalities
☐*Ears*: No abnormalities; ☐Debris (mild / mod / sev) (AU / AD / AS)
☐*Oral cavity*: No abnormalities; ☐Tarter (mild / mod/ sev); ☐Gingivitis
☐*Lymph nodes*: Small, symmetrical, smooth, and soft
☐*Abdomen*: Soft, non-painful, no fluid-wave, organomegaly, or masses
☐*Mammary Chain*: No abnormalities
☐*Penis/ Vulva*: No abnormalities
☐*Skin*: No alopecia, masses, erythema, other lesions, or ectoparasites
☐*Neuro*: No paresis, ataxia, or postural deficits, normal PLR and mentation
☐*MS*: Adequate and symmetrical muscling, no overt lameness
☐*Rectal*: No abnormalities, normal colored feces on glove

Labwork:

Other Diagnostics:
Blood Pressure:

Problem List:

Plan:

Case No._____

Patient	Age	Sex	Breed	Weight
	DOB:	Mn / Mi Fs / Fi	Color:	kg

Owner	Primary Veterinarian	Admit Date/ Time
Name: Phone:	Name: Phone:	Date: Time: AM / PM

- **Presenting Complaint**:_____
  _____
  _____

- **Medical Hx**:_____
  _____
  _____

- **When/ where obtained**:   Date:_____ ;   ☐Breeder, ☐Shelter, Other:_____

Drug/ Suppl.	Amount	Dose (mg/kg)	Route	Frequency	Date Started

- **Vaccine status – Dog**: ☐Rab ☐Parv ☐Dist ☐Aden; ☐Para ☐Lep ☐Bord ☐Influ ☐Lyme
- **Vaccine status – Cat**: ☐Rab ☐Herp ☐Cali ☐Pan ☐FeLV[kittens]; ☐FIV ☐Chlam ☐Bord
- **Heartworm / Flea & Tick / Intestinal Parasites**:
  - *Last Heartworm Test*: Date:_____, ☐IDK; Test Results: ☐Pos, ☐Neg, ☐IDK
  - *Monthly heartworm preventative*:   ☐no ☐yes, Product:_____
  - *Monthly flea & tick preventative*:   ☐no ☐yes, Product:_____
  - *Monthly dewormer*:   ☐no ☐yes, Product:_____
- **Surgical Hx**:   ☐Spay/Neuter; Date:_____; Other:_____
- **Environment**: ☐Indoor, ☐Outdoor, Time spent outdoors/ Other:_____
- **Housemates**: Dogs:____ Cats:____ Other:_____
- **Diet**: ☐Wet, ☐Dry; Brand/ Amt.:_____

Appetite	☐Normal, ☐↑, ☐↓
Weight	☐Normal, ☐↑, ☐↓; Past Wt.:_____ kg; Date:_____; Δ:_____
Thirst	☐Normal, ☐↑, ☐↓
Urination	☐Normal, ☐↑, ☐↓, ☐Blood, ☐Strain
Defecation	☐Normal, ☐↑, ☐↓, ☐Blood, ☐Strain, ☐Diarrhea, ☐Mucus
Discharge	☐No, ☐Yes; Onset/ Describe:
Cough/ Sneeze	☐No, ☐Yes; Onset/ Describe:
Vomit	☐No, ☐Yes; Onset/ Describe:
Respiration	☐Normal, ☐↑ Rate, ☐↑ Effort
Energy level	☐Normal, ☐Lethargic, ☐Exercise intolerance

- **Travel Hx**: ☐None, Other:_____
- **Exposure to**: ☐Standing water, ☐Wildlife, ☐Board/daycare, ☐Dog park, ☐Groomer
- **Adverse reactions to food/ meds**: ☐None, Other:_____
- Can give oral meds: ☐no ☐yes; Helpful Tricks:_____

Physical Exam:

T: *P:*   *R:*   *Wt.:*   *BCS:*   *Pain:*   *CRT:*

☐*CV*: Regular rhythm, no murmur, normokinetic and synchronous pulses
☐*Resp*: Normal BV sounds/ effort, normal tracheal sounds/ palpation
☐*Attitude*: Bright, alert, and responsive
☐*Hydration/ Perfusion*: MM pink and moist with a CRT of 1-2 sec
☐*Eyes*: No abnormalities
☐*Nose*: No abnormalities
☐*Ears*: No abnormalities; ☐Debris (mild / mod / sev) (AU / AD / AS)
☐*Oral cavity*: No abnormalities; ☐Tarter (mild / mod/ sev); ☐Gingivitis
☐*Lymph nodes*: Small, symmetrical, smooth, and soft
☐*Abdomen*: Soft, non-painful, no fluid-wave, organomegaly, or masses
☐*Mammary Chain*: No abnormalities
☐*Penis/ Vulva*: No abnormalities
☐*Skin*: No alopecia, masses, erythema, other lesions, or ectoparasites
☐*Neuro*: No paresis, ataxia, or postural deficits, normal PLR and mentation
☐*MS*: Adequate and symmetrical muscling, no overt lameness
☐*Rectal*: No abnormalities, normal colored feces on glove

Labwork:

Other Diagnostics:
Blood Pressure:

Problem List:

Plan:

Patient	Age	Sex	Breed	Weight
	DOB:	Mn / Mi Fs / Fi	Color:	kg

Owner		Primary Veterinarian	Admit Date/ Time
Name: Phone:		Name: Phone:	Date: Time: AM / PM

• **Presenting Complaint**:_____
_____
_____
_____

• **Medical Hx**:_____
_____
_____

• **When/ where obtained**:   Date:_____; ☐Breeder, ☐Shelter, Other:_____

Drug/ Suppl.	Amount	Dose (mg/kg)	Route	Frequency	Date Started

• **Vaccine status – Dog**: ☐Rab ☐Parv ☐Dist ☐Aden; ☐Para ☐Lep ☐Bord ☐Influ ☐Lyme
• **Vaccine status – Cat**: ☐Rab ☐Herp ☐Cali ☐Pan ☐FeLV[kittens]; ☐FIV ☐Chlam ☐Bord
• **Heartworm / Flea & Tick / Intestinal Parasites**:
  ○ *Last Heartworm Test*: Date:_____, ☐IDK; Test Results: ☐Pos, ☐Neg, ☐IDK
  ○ *Monthly heartworm preventative*: ☐no ☐yes, Product:_____
  ○ *Monthly flea & tick preventative*: ☐no ☐yes, Product:_____
  ○ *Monthly dewormer*:   ☐no ☐yes, Product:_____
• **Surgical Hx**: ☐Spay/Neuter; Date:_____; Other:_____
• **Environment**: ☐Indoor, ☐Outdoor, Time spent outdoors/ Other:_____
• **Housemates**: Dogs:_____ Cats:_____ Other:_____
• **Diet**: ☐Wet, ☐Dry; Brand/ Amt.:_____

Appetite	☐Normal, ☐↑, ☐↓
Weight	☐Normal, ☐↑, ☐↓; Past Wt.:_____ kg; Date:_____; Δ:_____
Thirst	☐Normal, ☐↑, ☐↓
Urination	☐Normal, ☐↑, ☐↓, ☐Blood, ☐Strain
Defecation	☐Normal, ☐↑, ☐↓, ☐Blood, ☐Strain, ☐Diarrhea, ☐Mucus
Discharge	☐No, ☐Yes; Onset/ Describe:
Cough/ Sneeze	☐No, ☐Yes; Onset/ Describe:
Vomit	☐No, ☐Yes; Onset/ Describe:
Respiration	☐Normal, ☐↑ Rate, ☐↑ Effort
Energy level	☐Normal, ☐Lethargic, ☐Exercise intolerance

• **Travel Hx**: ☐None, Other:_____
• **Exposure to**: ☐Standing water, ☐Wildlife, ☐Board/daycare, ☐Dog park, ☐Groomer
• **Adverse reactions to food/ meds**: ☐None, Other:_____
• Can give oral meds: ☐no ☐yes; Helpful Tricks:_____

Physical Exam:

T: *P:* *R:* *Wt.:* *BCS:* *Pain:* *CRT:*

☐*CV*: Regular rhythm, no murmur, normokinetic and synchronous pulses
☐*Resp*: Normal BV sounds/ effort, normal tracheal sounds/ palpation
☐*Attitude*: Bright, alert, and responsive
☐*Hydration/ Perfusion*: MM pink and moist with a CRT of 1-2 sec
☐*Eyes*: No abnormalities
☐*Nose*: No abnormalities
☐*Ears*: No abnormalities; ☐Debris (mild / mod / sev) (AU / AD / AS)
☐*Oral cavity*: No abnormalities; ☐Tarter (mild / mod/ sev); ☐Gingivitis
☐*Lymph nodes*: Small, symmetrical, smooth, and soft
☐*Abdomen*: Soft, non-painful, no fluid-wave, organomegaly, or masses
☐*Mammary Chain*: No abnormalities
☐*Penis/ Vulva*: No abnormalities
☐*Skin*: No alopecia, masses, erythema, other lesions, or ectoparasites
☐*Neuro*: No paresis, ataxia, or postural deficits, normal PLR and mentation
☐*MS*: Adequate and symmetrical muscling, no overt lameness
☐*Rectal*: No abnormalities, normal colored feces on glove

Labwork:

Other Diagnostics:
Blood Pressure:

Problem List:

Plan:

Case No._____

Patient	Age	Sex	Breed	Weight
	DOB:	Mn / Mi Fs / Fi	Color:	kg

Owner	Primary Veterinarian	Admit Date/ Time
Name: Phone:	Name: Phone:	Date: Time: AM / PM

• **Presenting Complaint**:_____
_____
_____

• **Medical Hx**:_____
_____
_____

• **When/ where obtained**:   Date:_____; ☐Breeder, ☐Shelter, Other:_____

Drug/ Suppl.	Amount	Dose (mg/kg)	Route	Frequency	Date Started

• **Vaccine status – Dog**: ☐Rab ☐Parv ☐Dist ☐Aden; ☐Para ☐Lep ☐Bord ☐Influ ☐Lyme
• **Vaccine status – Cat**: ☐Rab ☐Herp ☐Cali ☐Pan ☐FeLV[kittens]; ☐FIV ☐Chlam ☐Bord
• **Heartworm / Flea & Tick / Intestinal Parasites**:
  ◦ *Last Heartworm Test*: Date:_____, ☐IDK; Test Results: ☐Pos, ☐Neg, ☐IDK
  ◦ *Monthly heartworm preventative*: ☐no ☐yes, Product:_____
  ◦ *Monthly flea & tick preventative*: ☐no ☐yes, Product:_____
  ◦ *Monthly dewormer*:   ☐no ☐yes, Product:_____
• **Surgical Hx**:   ☐Spay/Neuter; Date:_____; Other:_____
• **Environment**: ☐Indoor, ☐Outdoor, Time spent outdoors/ Other:_____
• **Housemates**: Dogs:_____ Cats:_____ Other:_____
• **Diet**: ☐Wet, ☐Dry; Brand/ Amt.:_____

Appetite	☐Normal, ☐↑, ☐↓
Weight	☐Normal, ☐↑, ☐↓; Past Wt.:_____ kg; Date:_____; Δ:_____
Thirst	☐Normal, ☐↑, ☐↓
Urination	☐Normal, ☐↑, ☐↓, ☐Blood, ☐Strain
Defecation	☐Normal, ☐↑, ☐↓, ☐Blood, ☐Strain, ☐Diarrhea, ☐Mucus
Discharge	☐No, ☐Yes; Onset/ Describe:
Cough/ Sneeze	☐No, ☐Yes; Onset/ Describe:
Vomit	☐No, ☐Yes; Onset/ Describe:
Respiration	☐Normal, ☐↑ Rate, ☐↑ Effort
Energy level	☐Normal, ☐Lethargic, ☐Exercise intolerance

• **Travel Hx**: ☐None, Other:_____
• **Exposure to**: ☐Standing water, ☐Wildlife, ☐Board/daycare, ☐Dog park, ☐Groomer
• **Adverse reactions to food/ meds**: ☐None, Other:_____
• Can give oral meds: ☐no ☐yes; Helpful Tricks:_____

Physical Exam:

T: *P:* *R:* *Wt.:* *BCS:* *Pain:* *CRT:*

☐*CV*: Regular rhythm, no murmur, normokinetic and synchronous pulses
☐*Resp*: Normal BV sounds/ effort, normal tracheal sounds/ palpation
☐*Attitude*: Bright, alert, and responsive
☐*Hydration/ Perfusion*: MM pink and moist with a CRT of 1-2 sec
☐*Eyes*: No abnormalities
☐*Nose*: No abnormalities
☐*Ears*: No abnormalities; ☐Debris (mild / mod / sev) (AU / AD / AS)
☐*Oral cavity*: No abnormalities; ☐Tarter (mild / mod/ sev); ☐Gingivitis
☐*Lymph nodes*: Small, symmetrical, smooth, and soft
☐*Abdomen*: Soft, non-painful, no fluid-wave, organomegaly, or masses
☐*Mammary Chain*: No abnormalities
☐*Penis/ Vulva*: No abnormalities
☐*Skin*: No alopecia, masses, erythema, other lesions, or ectoparasites
☐*Neuro*: No paresis, ataxia, or postural deficits, normal PLR and mentation
☐*MS*: Adequate and symmetrical muscling, no overt lameness
☐*Rectal*: No abnormalities, normal colored feces on glove

Labwork:

Other Diagnostics:
Blood Pressure:

Problem List:

Plan:

Case No._____

Patient	Age	Sex	Breed	Weight
	DOB:	Mn / Mi Fs / Fi	Color:	kg

Owner	Primary Veterinarian	Admit Date/ Time
Name: Phone:	Name: Phone:	Date: Time: AM / PM

• **Presenting Complaint**:_____
_____
_____
_____

• **Medical Hx**:_____
_____
_____

• **When/ where obtained**:   Date:_____; □Breeder, □Shelter, Other:_____

Drug/ Suppl.	Amount	Dose (mg/kg)	Route	Frequency	Date Started

• **Vaccine status – Dog**: □Rab □Parv □Dist □Aden; □Para □Lep □Bord □Influ □Lyme
• **Vaccine status – Cat**: □Rab □Herp □Cali □Pan □FeLV[kittens]; □FIV □Chlam □Bord
• **Heartworm / Flea & Tick / Intestinal Parasites**:
   ◦ *Last Heartworm Test*: Date:_____, □IDK; Test Results: □Pos, □Neg, □IDK
   ◦ *Monthly heartworm preventative*: □no □yes, Product:_____
   ◦ *Monthly flea & tick preventative*: □no □yes, Product:_____
   ◦ *Monthly dewormer*:   □no □yes, Product:_____
• **Surgical Hx**:   □Spay/Neuter; Date:_____; Other:_____
• **Environment**: □Indoor, □Outdoor, Time spent outdoors/ Other:_____
• **Housemates**: Dogs:_____ Cats:_____ Other:_____
• **Diet**: □Wet, □Dry; Brand/ Amt.:_____

Appetite	□Normal, □↑, □↓
Weight	□Normal, □↑, □↓; Past Wt.:_____ kg; Date:_____; Δ:_____
Thirst	□Normal, □↑, □↓
Urination	□Normal, □↑, □↓, □Blood, □Strain
Defecation	□Normal, □↑, □↓, □Blood, □Strain, □Diarrhea, □Mucus
Discharge	□No, □Yes; Onset/ Describe:
Cough/ Sneeze	□No, □Yes; Onset/ Describe:
Vomit	□No, □Yes; Onset/ Describe:
Respiration	□Normal, □↑ Rate, □↑ Effort
Energy level	□Normal, □Lethargic, □Exercise intolerance

• **Travel Hx**: □None, Other:_____
• **Exposure to**: □Standing water, □Wildlife, □Board/daycare, □Dog park, □Groomer
• **Adverse reactions to food/ meds**: □None, Other:_____
• Can give oral meds: □no □yes; Helpful Tricks:_____

Physical Exam:

T: P: R: Wt.: BCS: Pain: CRT:

☐*CV*: Regular rhythm, no murmur, normokinetic and synchronous pulses
☐*Resp*: Normal BV sounds/ effort, normal tracheal sounds/ palpation
☐*Attitude*: Bright, alert, and responsive
☐*Hydration/ Perfusion*: MM pink and moist with a CRT of 1-2 sec
☐*Eyes*: No abnormalities
☐*Nose*: No abnormalities
☐*Ears*: No abnormalities; ☐Debris (mild / mod / sev) (AU / AD / AS)
☐*Oral cavity*: No abnormalities; ☐Tarter (mild / mod/ sev); ☐Gingivitis
☐*Lymph nodes*: Small, symmetrical, smooth, and soft
☐*Abdomen*: Soft, non-painful, no fluid-wave, organomegaly, or masses
☐*Mammary Chain*: No abnormalities
☐*Penis/ Vulva*: No abnormalities
☐*Skin*: No alopecia, masses, erythema, other lesions, or ectoparasites
☐*Neuro*: No paresis, ataxia, or postural deficits, normal PLR and mentation
☐*MS*: Adequate and symmetrical muscling, no overt lameness
☐*Rectal*: No abnormalities, normal colored feces on glove

Labwork:

Other Diagnostics:
Blood Pressure:

Problem List:

Plan:

Patient	Age	Sex	Breed	Weight
	DOB:	Mn / Mi Fs / Fi	Color:	kg

Owner	Primary Veterinarian	Admit Date/ Time
Name: Phone:	Name: Phone:	Date: Time: AM / PM

• **Presenting Complaint**:_____
_____
_____

• **Medical Hx**:_____
_____
_____

• **When/ where obtained**:   Date:_____; □Breeder, □Shelter, Other:_____

Drug/ Suppl.	Amount	Dose (mg/kg)	Route	Frequency	Date Started

• **Vaccine status – Dog**: □Rab □Parv □Dist □Aden; □Para □Lep □Bord □Influ □Lyme
• **Vaccine status – Cat**: □Rab □Herp □Cali □Pan □FeLV[kittens]; □FIV □Chlam □Bord
• **Heartworm / Flea & Tick / Intestinal Parasites**:
  ◦ *Last Heartworm Test*: Date:_____, □IDK; Test Results: □Pos, □Neg, □IDK
  ◦ *Monthly heartworm preventative*: □no □yes, Product:_____
  ◦ *Monthly flea & tick preventative*: □no □yes, Product:_____
  ◦ *Monthly dewormer*: □no □yes, Product:_____
• **Surgical Hx**:   □Spay/Neuter; Date:_____; Other:_____
• **Environment**: □Indoor, □Outdoor, Time spent outdoors/ Other:_____
• **Housemates**: Dogs:_____ Cats:_____ Other:_____
• **Diet**: □Wet, □Dry; Brand/ Amt.:_____

Appetite	□Normal, □↑, □↓
Weight	□Normal, □↑, □↓; Past Wt.:_____ kg; Date:_____; Δ:_____
Thirst	□Normal, □↑, □↓
Urination	□Normal, □↑, □↓, □Blood, □Strain
Defecation	□Normal, □↑, □↓, □Blood, □Strain, □Diarrhea, □Mucus
Discharge	□No, □Yes; Onset/ Describe:
Cough/ Sneeze	□No, □Yes; Onset/ Describe:
Vomit	□No, □Yes; Onset/ Describe:
Respiration	□Normal, □↑ Rate, □↑ Effort
Energy level	□Normal, □Lethargic, □Exercise intolerance

• **Travel Hx**: □None, Other:_____
• **Exposure to**: □Standing water, □Wildlife, □Board/daycare, □Dog park, □Groomer
• **Adverse reactions to food/ meds**: □None, Other:_____
• Can give oral meds: □no □yes; Helpful Tricks:_____

Physical Exam:

T: P: R: Wt.:   BCS: Pain: CRT:

☐*CV*: Regular rhythm, no murmur, normokinetic and synchronous pulses
☐*Resp*: Normal BV sounds/ effort, normal tracheal sounds/ palpation
☐*Attitude*: Bright, alert, and responsive
☐*Hydration/ Perfusion*: MM pink and moist with a CRT of 1-2 sec
☐*Eyes*: No abnormalities
☐*Nose*: No abnormalities
☐*Ears*: No abnormalities; ☐Debris (mild / mod / sev) (AU / AD / AS)
☐*Oral cavity*: No abnormalities; ☐Tarter (mild / mod/ sev); ☐Gingivitis
☐*Lymph nodes*: Small, symmetrical, smooth, and soft
☐*Abdomen*: Soft, non-painful, no fluid-wave, organomegaly, or masses
☐*Mammary Chain*: No abnormalities
☐*Penis/ Vulva*: No abnormalities
☐*Skin*: No alopecia, masses, erythema, other lesions, or ectoparasites
☐*Neuro*: No paresis, ataxia, or postural deficits, normal PLR and mentation
☐*MS*: Adequate and symmetrical muscling, no overt lameness
☐*Rectal*: No abnormalities, normal colored feces on glove

Labwork:

Other Diagnostics:
Blood Pressure:

Problem List:

Plan:

Case No._____

Patient	Age	Sex	Breed	Weight
	DOB:	Mn / Mi Fs / Fi	Color:	kg

Owner	Primary Veterinarian	Admit Date/ Time
Name: Phone:	Name: Phone:	Date: Time: AM / PM

- **Presenting Complaint**:_____
_____
_____

- **Medical Hx**:_____
_____
_____

- **When/ where obtained**:   Date:_____; □Breeder, □Shelter, Other:_____

Drug/ Suppl.	Amount	Dose (mg/kg)	Route	Frequency	Date Started

- **Vaccine status – Dog**: □Rab □Parv □Dist □Aden; □Para □Lep □Bord □Influ □Lyme
- **Vaccine status – Cat**: □Rab □Herp □Cali □Pan □FeLV[kittens]; □FIV □Chlam □Bord
- **Heartworm / Flea & Tick / Intestinal Parasites**:
  ◦ *Last Heartworm Test*: Date:_____, □IDK; Test Results: □Pos, □Neg, □IDK
  ◦ *Monthly heartworm preventative*: □no □yes, Product:_____
  ◦ *Monthly flea & tick preventative*: □no □yes, Product:_____
  ◦ *Monthly dewormer*: □no □yes, Product:_____
- **Surgical Hx**: □Spay/Neuter; Date:_____; Other:_____
- **Environment**: □Indoor, □Outdoor, Time spent outdoors/ Other:_____
- **Housemates**: Dogs:_____ Cats:_____ Other:_____
- **Diet**: □Wet, □Dry; Brand/ Amt.:_____

Appetite	□Normal, □↑, □↓
Weight	□Normal, □↑, □↓; Past Wt.:_____ kg; Date:_____; Δ:_____
Thirst	□Normal, □↑, □↓
Urination	□Normal, □↑, □↓, □Blood, □Strain
Defecation	□Normal, □↑, □↓, □Blood, □Strain, □Diarrhea, □Mucus
Discharge	□No, □Yes; Onset/ Describe:
Cough/ Sneeze	□No, □Yes; Onset/ Describe:
Vomit	□No, □Yes; Onset/ Describe:
Respiration	□Normal, □↑ Rate, □↑ Effort
Energy level	□Normal, □Lethargic, □Exercise intolerance

- **Travel Hx**: □None, Other:_____
- **Exposure to**: □Standing water, □Wildlife, □Board/daycare, □Dog park, □Groomer
- **Adverse reactions to food/ meds**: □None, Other:_____
- Can give oral meds: □no □yes; Helpful Tricks:_____

Physical Exam:

T: *P:*   *R:*   *Wt.:*   *BCS:*   *Pain:*   *CRT:*

☐*CV*: Regular rhythm, no murmur, normokinetic and synchronous pulses
☐*Resp*: Normal BV sounds/ effort, normal tracheal sounds/ palpation
☐*Attitude*: Bright, alert, and responsive
☐*Hydration/ Perfusion*: MM pink and moist with a CRT of 1-2 sec
☐*Eyes*: No abnormalities
☐*Nose*: No abnormalities
☐*Ears*: No abnormalities; ☐Debris (mild / mod / sev) (AU / AD / AS)
☐*Oral cavity*: No abnormalities; ☐Tarter (mild / mod/ sev); ☐Gingivitis
☐*Lymph nodes*: Small, symmetrical, smooth, and soft
☐*Abdomen*: Soft, non-painful, no fluid-wave, organomegaly, or masses
☐*Mammary Chain*: No abnormalities
☐*Penis/ Vulva*: No abnormalities
☐*Skin*: No alopecia, masses, erythema, other lesions, or ectoparasites
☐*Neuro*: No paresis, ataxia, or postural deficits, normal PLR and mentation
☐*MS*: Adequate and symmetrical muscling, no overt lameness
☐*Rectal*: No abnormalities, normal colored feces on glove

Labwork:

Other Diagnostics:
Blood Pressure:

Problem List:

Plan:

Case No._____

Patient	Age	Sex	Breed	Weight
	DOB:	Mn / Mi Fs / Fi	Color:	kg

Owner	Primary Veterinarian	Admit Date/ Time
Name: Phone:	Name: Phone:	Date: Time: AM / PM

• **Presenting Complaint**:_____

_____

_____

• **Medical Hx**:_____

_____

_____

• **When/ where obtained**:   Date:_____; □Breeder, □Shelter, Other:_____

Drug/ Suppl.	Amount	Dose (mg/kg)	Route	Frequency	Date Started

• **Vaccine status – Dog**: □Rab □Parv □Dist □Aden; □Para □Lep □Bord □Influ □Lyme
• **Vaccine status – Cat**: □Rab □Herp □Cali □Pan □FeLV[kittens]; □FIV □Chlam □Bord
• **Heartworm / Flea & Tick / Intestinal Parasites**:
   ◦ *Last Heartworm Test*: Date:_____, □IDK;   Test Results: □Pos, □Neg, □IDK
   ◦ *Monthly heartworm preventative*: □no □yes,   Product:_____
   ◦ *Monthly flea & tick preventative*: □no □yes,   Product:_____
   ◦ *Monthly dewormer*: □no □yes,   Product:_____
• **Surgical Hx**:   □Spay/Neuter; Date:_____;   Other:_____
• **Environment**: □Indoor, □Outdoor, Time spent outdoors/ Other:_____
• **Housemates**: Dogs:_____ Cats:_____ Other:_____
• **Diet**: □Wet, □Dry; Brand/ Amt.:_____

Appetite	□Normal, □↑, □↓
Weight	□Normal, □↑, □↓; Past Wt.:_____ kg; Date:_____; Δ:_____
Thirst	□Normal, □↑, □↓
Urination	□Normal, □↑, □↓, □Blood, □Strain
Defecation	□Normal, □↑, □↓, □Blood, □Strain, □Diarrhea, □Mucus
Discharge	□No, □Yes; Onset/ Describe:
Cough/ Sneeze	□No, □Yes; Onset/ Describe:
Vomit	□No, □Yes; Onset/ Describe:
Respiration	□Normal, □↑ Rate, □↑ Effort
Energy level	□Normal, □Lethargic, □Exercise intolerance

• **Travel Hx**: □None, Other:_____
• **Exposure to**: □Standing water, □Wildlife, □Board/daycare, □Dog park, □Groomer
• **Adverse reactions to food/ meds**: □None, Other:_____
• Can give oral meds: □no □yes; Helpful Tricks:_____

Physical Exam:

T: P: R: Wt.:   BCS: Pain: CRT:

☐*CV*: Regular rhythm, no murmur, normokinetic and synchronous pulses
☐*Resp*: Normal BV sounds/ effort, normal tracheal sounds/ palpation
☐*Attitude*: Bright, alert, and responsive
☐*Hydration/ Perfusion*: MM pink and moist with a CRT of 1-2 sec
☐*Eyes*: No abnormalities
☐*Nose*: No abnormalities
☐*Ears*: No abnormalities; ☐Debris (mild / mod / sev) (AU / AD / AS)
☐*Oral cavity*: No abnormalities; ☐Tarter (mild / mod/ sev); ☐Gingivitis
☐*Lymph nodes*: Small, symmetrical, smooth, and soft
☐*Abdomen*: Soft, non-painful, no fluid-wave, organomegaly, or masses
☐*Mammary Chain*: No abnormalities
☐*Penis/ Vulva*: No abnormalities
☐*Skin*: No alopecia, masses, erythema, other lesions, or ectoparasites
☐*Neuro*: No paresis, ataxia, or postural deficits, normal PLR and mentation
☐*MS*: Adequate and symmetrical muscling, no overt lameness
☐*Rectal*: No abnormalities, normal colored feces on glove

Labwork:

Other Diagnostics:
Blood Pressure:

Problem List:

Plan:

Patient	Age	Sex	Breed	Weight
	DOB:	Mn / Mi Fs / Fi	Color:	kg

Owner	Primary Veterinarian	Admit Date/ Time
Name: Phone:	Name: Phone:	Date: Time: AM / PM

• **Presenting Complaint**:_____
_____
_____

• **Medical Hx**:_____
_____
_____

• **When/ where obtained**: Date:_____ ; ☐Breeder, ☐Shelter, Other:_____

Drug/ Suppl.	Amount	Dose (mg/kg)	Route	Frequency	Date Started

• **Vaccine status – Dog**: ☐Rab ☐Parv ☐Dist ☐Aden; ☐Para ☐Lep ☐Bord ☐Influ ☐Lyme
• **Vaccine status – Cat**: ☐Rab ☐Herp ☐Cali ☐Pan ☐FeLV[kittens]; ☐FIV ☐Chlam ☐Bord
• **Heartworm / Flea & Tick / Intestinal Parasites**:
   ◦ *Last Heartworm Test*: Date:_____, ☐IDK; Test Results: ☐Pos, ☐Neg, ☐IDK
   ◦ *Monthly heartworm preventative*: ☐no ☐yes, Product:_____
   ◦ *Monthly flea & tick preventative*: ☐no ☐yes, Product:_____
   ◦ *Monthly dewormer*: ☐no ☐yes, Product:_____
• **Surgical Hx**: ☐Spay/Neuter; Date:_____; Other:_____
• **Environment**: ☐Indoor, ☐Outdoor, Time spent outdoors/ Other:_____
• **Housemates**: Dogs:_____ Cats:_____ Other:_____
• **Diet**: ☐Wet, ☐Dry; Brand/ Amt.:_____

Appetite	☐Normal, ☐↑, ☐↓
Weight	☐Normal, ☐↑, ☐↓; Past Wt.:_____ kg; Date:_____; Δ:_____
Thirst	☐Normal, ☐↑, ☐↓
Urination	☐Normal, ☐↑, ☐↓, ☐Blood, ☐Strain
Defecation	☐Normal, ☐↑, ☐↓, ☐Blood, ☐Strain, ☐Diarrhea, ☐Mucus
Discharge	☐No, ☐Yes; Onset/ Describe:
Cough/ Sneeze	☐No, ☐Yes; Onset/ Describe:
Vomit	☐No, ☐Yes; Onset/ Describe:
Respiration	☐Normal, ☐↑ Rate, ☐↑ Effort
Energy level	☐Normal, ☐Lethargic, ☐Exercise intolerance

• **Travel Hx**: ☐None, Other:_____
• **Exposure to**: ☐Standing water, ☐Wildlife, ☐Board/daycare, ☐Dog park, ☐Groomer
• **Adverse reactions to food/ meds**: ☐None, Other:_____
• Can give oral meds: ☐no ☐yes; Helpful Tricks:_____

Physical Exam:

T: P: R: Wt.:   BCS: Pain: CRT:

☐*CV*: Regular rhythm, no murmur, normokinetic and synchronous pulses
☐*Resp*: Normal BV sounds/ effort, normal tracheal sounds/ palpation
☐*Attitude*: Bright, alert, and responsive
☐*Hydration/ Perfusion*: MM pink and moist with a CRT of 1-2 sec
☐*Eyes*: No abnormalities
☐*Nose*: No abnormalities
☐*Ears*: No abnormalities; ☐Debris (mild / mod / sev) (AU / AD / AS)
☐*Oral cavity*: No abnormalities; ☐Tarter (mild / mod/ sev); ☐Gingivitis
☐*Lymph nodes*: Small, symmetrical, smooth, and soft
☐*Abdomen*: Soft, non-painful, no fluid-wave, organomegaly, or masses
☐*Mammary Chain*: No abnormalities
☐*Penis/ Vulva*: No abnormalities
☐*Skin*: No alopecia, masses, erythema, other lesions, or ectoparasites
☐*Neuro*: No paresis, ataxia, or postural deficits, normal PLR and mentation
☐*MS*: Adequate and symmetrical muscling, no overt lameness
☐*Rectal*: No abnormalities, normal colored feces on glove

Labwork:

Other Diagnostics:
Blood Pressure:

Problem List:

Plan:

Case No._____

Patient	Age	Sex	Breed	Weight
	DOB:	Mn / Mi Fs / Fi	Color:	kg

Owner	Primary Veterinarian	Admit Date/ Time
Name: Phone:	Name: Phone:	Date: Time: AM / PM

• **Presenting Complaint**:_____
_____
_____

• **Medical Hx**:_____
_____
_____

• **When/ where obtained**: Date:_____ ; ☐Breeder, ☐Shelter, Other:_____

Drug/ Suppl.	Amount	Dose (mg/kg)	Route	Frequency	Date Started

• **Vaccine status – Dog**: ☐Rab ☐Parv ☐Dist ☐Aden; ☐Para ☐Lep ☐Bord ☐Influ ☐Lyme
• **Vaccine status – Cat**: ☐Rab ☐Herp ☐Cali ☐Pan ☐FeLV[kittens]; ☐FIV ☐Chlam ☐Bord
• **Heartworm / Flea & Tick / Intestinal Parasites**:
   ◦ *Last Heartworm Test*: Date:_____, ☐IDK; Test Results: ☐Pos, ☐Neg, ☐IDK
   ◦ *Monthly heartworm preventative*: ☐no ☐yes, Product:_____
   ◦ *Monthly flea & tick preventative*: ☐no ☐yes, Product:_____
   ◦ *Monthly dewormer*:   ☐no ☐yes, Product:_____
• **Surgical Hx**: ☐Spay/Neuter; Date:_____; Other:_____
• **Environment**: ☐Indoor, ☐Outdoor, Time spent outdoors/ Other:_____
• **Housemates**: Dogs:_____ Cats:_____ Other:_____
• **Diet**: ☐Wet, ☐Dry; Brand/ Amt.:_____

Appetite	☐Normal, ☐↑, ☐↓
Weight	☐Normal, ☐↑, ☐↓; Past Wt.:_____ kg; Date:_____; Δ:_____
Thirst	☐Normal, ☐↑, ☐↓
Urination	☐Normal, ☐↑, ☐↓, ☐Blood, ☐Strain
Defecation	☐Normal, ☐↑, ☐↓, ☐Blood, ☐Strain, ☐Diarrhea, ☐Mucus
Discharge	☐No, ☐Yes; Onset/ Describe:
Cough/ Sneeze	☐No, ☐Yes; Onset/ Describe:
Vomit	☐No, ☐Yes; Onset/ Describe:
Respiration	☐Normal, ☐↑ Rate, ☐↑ Effort
Energy level	☐Normal, ☐Lethargic, ☐Exercise intolerance

• **Travel Hx**: ☐None, Other:_____
• **Exposure to**: ☐Standing water, ☐Wildlife, ☐Board/daycare, ☐Dog park, ☐Groomer
• **Adverse reactions to food/ meds**: ☐None, Other:_____
• Can give oral meds: ☐no ☐yes; Helpful Tricks:_____

Physical Exam:

T: P: R: Wt.:   BCS: Pain: CRT:

☐*CV*: Regular rhythm, no murmur, normokinetic and synchronous pulses
☐*Resp*: Normal BV sounds/ effort, normal tracheal sounds/ palpation
☐*Attitude*: Bright, alert, and responsive
☐*Hydration/ Perfusion*: MM pink and moist with a CRT of 1-2 sec
☐*Eyes*: No abnormalities
☐*Nose*: No abnormalities
☐*Ears*: No abnormalities; ☐Debris (mild / mod / sev) (AU / AD / AS)
☐*Oral cavity*: No abnormalities; ☐Tarter (mild / mod/ sev); ☐Gingivitis
☐*Lymph nodes*: Small, symmetrical, smooth, and soft
☐*Abdomen*: Soft, non-painful, no fluid-wave, organomegaly, or masses
☐*Mammary Chain*: No abnormalities
☐*Penis/ Vulva*: No abnormalities
☐*Skin*: No alopecia, masses, erythema, other lesions, or ectoparasites
☐*Neuro*: No paresis, ataxia, or postural deficits, normal PLR and mentation
☐*MS*: Adequate and symmetrical muscling, no overt lameness
☐*Rectal*: No abnormalities, normal colored feces on glove

Labwork:

Other Diagnostics:
Blood Pressure:

Problem List:

Plan:

Case No._____

Patient	Age	Sex	Breed	Weight
	DOB:	Mn / Mi Fs / Fi	Color:	kg

Owner	Primary Veterinarian	Admit Date/ Time
Name: Phone:	Name: Phone:	Date: Time: AM / PM

• **Presenting Complaint**:_____
_____
_____

• **Medical Hx**:_____
_____
_____

• **When/ where obtained**:   Date:_____; ☐Breeder, ☐Shelter, Other:_____

Drug/ Suppl.	Amount	Dose (mg/kg)	Route	Frequency	Date Started

• **Vaccine status – Dog**: ☐Rab ☐Parv ☐Dist ☐Aden; ☐Para ☐Lep ☐Bord ☐Influ ☐Lyme
• **Vaccine status – Cat**: ☐Rab ☐Herp ☐Cali ☐Pan ☐FeLV[kittens]; ☐FIV ☐Chlam ☐Bord
• **Heartworm / Flea & Tick / Intestinal Parasites**:
   ○ *Last Heartworm Test*: Date:_____, ☐IDK;   Test Results: ☐Pos, ☐Neg, ☐IDK
   ○ *Monthly heartworm preventative*: ☐no ☐yes,   Product:_____
   ○ *Monthly flea & tick preventative*: ☐no ☐yes,   Product:_____
   ○ *Monthly dewormer*:   ☐no ☐yes,   Product:_____
• **Surgical Hx**:   ☐Spay/Neuter; Date:_____;   Other:_____
• **Environment**: ☐Indoor, ☐Outdoor, Time spent outdoors/ Other:_____
• **Housemates**: Dogs:_____ Cats:_____ Other:_____
• **Diet**: ☐Wet, ☐Dry; Brand/ Amt.:_____

Appetite	☐Normal, ☐↑, ☐↓
Weight	☐Normal, ☐↑, ☐↓; Past Wt.:_____ kg; Date:_____; Δ:_____
Thirst	☐Normal, ☐↑, ☐↓
Urination	☐Normal, ☐↑, ☐↓, ☐Blood, ☐Strain
Defecation	☐Normal, ☐↑, ☐↓, ☐Blood, ☐Strain, ☐Diarrhea, ☐Mucus
Discharge	☐No, ☐Yes; Onset/ Describe:
Cough/ Sneeze	☐No, ☐Yes; Onset/ Describe:
Vomit	☐No, ☐Yes; Onset/ Describe:
Respiration	☐Normal, ☐↑ Rate, ☐↑ Effort
Energy level	☐Normal, ☐Lethargic, ☐Exercise intolerance

• **Travel Hx**: ☐None, Other:_____
• **Exposure to**: ☐Standing water, ☐Wildlife, ☐Board/daycare, ☐Dog park, ☐Groomer
• **Adverse reactions to food/ meds**: ☐None, Other:_____
• **Can give oral meds**: ☐no ☐yes; Helpful Tricks:_____

Physical Exam:

T:　　　P:　　　R:　　　Wt.:　　　BCS:　　　Pain:　　　CRT:

☐*CV*: Regular rhythm, no murmur, normokinetic and synchronous pulses
☐*Resp*: Normal BV sounds/ effort, normal tracheal sounds/ palpation
☐*Attitude*: Bright, alert, and responsive
☐*Hydration/ Perfusion*: MM pink and moist with a CRT of 1-2 sec
☐*Eyes*: No abnormalities
☐*Nose*: No abnormalities
☐*Ears*: No abnormalities; ☐Debris (mild / mod / sev) (AU / AD / AS)
☐*Oral cavity*: No abnormalities; ☐Tarter (mild / mod/ sev); ☐Gingivitis
☐*Lymph nodes*: Small, symmetrical, smooth, and soft
☐*Abdomen*: Soft, non-painful, no fluid-wave, organomegaly, or masses
☐*Mammary Chain*: No abnormalities
☐*Penis/ Vulva*: No abnormalities
☐*Skin*: No alopecia, masses, erythema, other lesions, or ectoparasites
☐*Neuro*: No paresis, ataxia, or postural deficits, normal PLR and mentation
☐*MS*: Adequate and symmetrical muscling, no overt lameness
☐*Rectal*: No abnormalities, normal colored feces on glove

Labwork:

Other Diagnostics:
Blood Pressure:

Problem List:

Plan:

Case No._____

Patient	Age	Sex	Breed	Weight
	DOB:	Mn / Mi Fs / Fi	Color:	kg

Owner	Primary Veterinarian	Admit Date/ Time
Name: Phone:	Name: Phone:	Date: Time: AM / PM

• **Presenting Complaint**:_____

_____

_____

• **Medical Hx**:_____

_____

_____

• **When/ where obtained**: Date:_____; □Breeder, □Shelter, Other:_____

Drug/ Suppl.	Amount	Dose (mg/kg)	Route	Frequency	Date Started

• **Vaccine status – Dog**: □Rab □Parv □Dist □Aden; □Para □Lep □Bord □Influ □Lyme
• **Vaccine status – Cat**: □Rab □Herp □Cali □Pan □FeLV[kittens]; □FIV □Chlam □Bord
• **Heartworm / Flea & Tick / Intestinal Parasites**:
   ◦ *Last Heartworm Test*: Date:_____, □IDK; Test Results: □Pos, □Neg, □IDK
   ◦ *Monthly heartworm preventative*: □no □yes, Product:_____
   ◦ *Monthly flea & tick preventative*: □no □yes, Product:_____
   ◦ *Monthly dewormer*:   □no □yes, Product:_____
• **Surgical Hx**: □Spay/Neuter; Date:_____; Other:_____
• **Environment**: □Indoor, □Outdoor, Time spent outdoors/ Other:_____
• **Housemates**: Dogs:_____ Cats:_____ Other:_____
• **Diet**: □Wet, □Dry; Brand/ Amt.:_____

Appetite	□Normal, □↑, □↓
Weight	□Normal, □↑, □↓; Past Wt.:_____ kg; Date:_____; Δ:_____
Thirst	□Normal, □↑, □↓
Urination	□Normal, □↑, □↓, □Blood, □Strain
Defecation	□Normal, □↑, □↓, □Blood, □Strain, □Diarrhea, □Mucus
Discharge	□No, □Yes; Onset/ Describe:
Cough/ Sneeze	□No, □Yes; Onset/ Describe:
Vomit	□No, □Yes; Onset/ Describe:
Respiration	□Normal, □↑ Rate, □↑ Effort
Energy level	□Normal, □Lethargic, □Exercise intolerance

• **Travel Hx**: □None, Other:_____
• **Exposure to**: □Standing water, □Wildlife, □Board/daycare, □Dog park, □Groomer
• **Adverse reactions to food/ meds**: □None, Other:_____
• Can give oral meds: □no □yes; Helpful Tricks:_____

Physical Exam:

T: *P:*   *R:*   *Wt.:*   *BCS:*   *Pain:*   *CRT:*

☐*CV*: Regular rhythm, no murmur, normokinetic and synchronous pulses
☐*Resp*: Normal BV sounds/ effort, normal tracheal sounds/ palpation
☐*Attitude*: Bright, alert, and responsive
☐*Hydration/ Perfusion*: MM pink and moist with a CRT of 1-2 sec
☐*Eyes*: No abnormalities
☐*Nose*: No abnormalities
☐*Ears*: No abnormalities; ☐Debris (mild / mod / sev) (AU / AD / AS)
☐*Oral cavity*: No abnormalities; ☐Tarter (mild / mod/ sev); ☐Gingivitis
☐*Lymph nodes*: Small, symmetrical, smooth, and soft
☐*Abdomen*: Soft, non-painful, no fluid-wave, organomegaly, or masses
☐*Mammary Chain*: No abnormalities
☐*Penis/ Vulva*: No abnormalities
☐*Skin*: No alopecia, masses, erythema, other lesions, or ectoparasites
☐*Neuro*: No paresis, ataxia, or postural deficits, normal PLR and mentation
☐*MS*: Adequate and symmetrical muscling, no overt lameness
☐*Rectal*: No abnormalities, normal colored feces on glove

Labwork:

Other Diagnostics:
Blood Pressure:

Problem List:

Plan:

Case No._____

Patient	Age	Sex	Breed		Weight
	DOB:	Mn / Mi Fs / Fi	Color:		kg

Owner		Primary Veterinarian	Admit Date/ Time
Name: Phone:		Name: Phone:	Date: Time: AM / PM

- **Presenting Complaint**:_____
  _____
  _____

- **Medical Hx**:_____
  _____
  _____

- **When/ where obtained**:   Date:_____;   □Breeder, □Shelter, Other:_____

Drug/ Suppl.	Amount	Dose (mg/kg)	Route	Frequency	Date Started

- **Vaccine status – Dog**: □Rab □Parv □Dist □Aden; □Para □Lep □Bord □Influ □Lyme
- **Vaccine status – Cat**: □Rab □Herp □Cali □Pan □FeLV[kittens]; □FIV □Chlam □Bord
- **Heartworm / Flea & Tick / Intestinal Parasites**:
  - *Last Heartworm Test*: Date:_____, □IDK; Test Results: □Pos, □Neg, □IDK
  - *Monthly heartworm preventative*:   □no □yes, Product:_____
  - *Monthly flea & tick preventative*:   □no □yes, Product:_____
  - *Monthly dewormer*:   □no □yes, Product:_____
- **Surgical Hx**:   □Spay/Neuter; Date:_____;   Other:_____
- **Environment**: □Indoor, □Outdoor, Time spent outdoors/ Other:_____
- **Housemates**: Dogs:_____ Cats:_____ Other:_____
- **Diet**: □Wet, □Dry; Brand/ Amt.:_____

Appetite	□Normal, □↑, □↓
Weight	□Normal, □↑, □↓; Past Wt.:_____ kg; Date:_____; Δ:_____
Thirst	□Normal, □↑, □↓
Urination	□Normal, □↑, □↓, □Blood, □Strain
Defecation	□Normal, □↑, □↓, □Blood, □Strain, □Diarrhea, □Mucus
Discharge	□No, □Yes; Onset/ Describe:
Cough/ Sneeze	□No, □Yes; Onset/ Describe:
Vomit	□No, □Yes; Onset/ Describe:
Respiration	□Normal, □↑ Rate, □↑ Effort
Energy level	□Normal, □Lethargic, □Exercise intolerance

- **Travel Hx**: □None, Other:_____
- **Exposure to**: □Standing water, □Wildlife, □Board/daycare, □Dog park, □Groomer
- **Adverse reactions to food/ meds**: □None, Other:_____
- Can give oral meds: □no □yes; Helpful Tricks:_____

Physical Exam:

T: P: R: Wt.:   BCS: Pain: CRT:

☐*CV*: Regular rhythm, no murmur, normokinetic and synchronous pulses
☐*Resp*: Normal BV sounds/ effort, normal tracheal sounds/ palpation
☐*Attitude*: Bright, alert, and responsive
☐*Hydration/ Perfusion*: MM pink and moist with a CRT of 1-2 sec
☐*Eyes*: No abnormalities
☐*Nose*: No abnormalities
☐*Ears*: No abnormalities; ☐Debris (mild / mod / sev) (AU / AD / AS)
☐*Oral cavity*: No abnormalities; ☐Tarter (mild / mod/ sev); ☐Gingivitis
☐*Lymph nodes*: Small, symmetrical, smooth, and soft
☐*Abdomen*: Soft, non-painful, no fluid-wave, organomegaly, or masses
☐*Mammary Chain*: No abnormalities
☐*Penis/ Vulva*: No abnormalities
☐*Skin*: No alopecia, masses, erythema, other lesions, or ectoparasites
☐*Neuro*: No paresis, ataxia, or postural deficits, normal PLR and mentation
☐*MS*: Adequate and symmetrical muscling, no overt lameness
☐*Rectal*: No abnormalities, normal colored feces on glove

Labwork:

Other Diagnostics:
Blood Pressure:

Problem List:

Plan:

Case No._____

Patient	Age	Sex	Breed	Weight
	DOB:	Mn / Mi Fs / Fi	Color:	kg

Owner	Primary Veterinarian	Admit Date/ Time
Name: Phone:	Name: Phone:	Date: Time: AM / PM

- **Presenting Complaint**:_____
  _____
  _____

- **Medical Hx**:_____
  _____
  _____

- **When/ where obtained**:   Date:_____ ; □Breeder, □Shelter, Other:_____

Drug/ Suppl.	Amount	Dose (mg/kg)	Route	Frequency	Date Started

- **Vaccine status – Dog**: □Rab □Parv □Dist □Aden; □Para □Lep □Bord □Influ □Lyme
- **Vaccine status – Cat**: □Rab □Herp □Cali □Pan □FeLV[kittens]; □FIV □Chlam □Bord
- **Heartworm / Flea & Tick / Intestinal Parasites**:
  - *Last Heartworm Test*: Date:_____, □IDK; Test Results: □Pos, □Neg, □IDK
  - *Monthly heartworm preventative*:   □no □yes, Product:_____
  - *Monthly flea & tick preventative*:   □no □yes, Product:_____
  - *Monthly dewormer*:   □no □yes, Product:_____
- **Surgical Hx**:   □Spay/Neuter; Date:_____ ; Other:_____
- **Environment**: □Indoor, □Outdoor, Time spent outdoors/ Other:_____
- **Housemates**: Dogs:_____ Cats:_____ Other:_____
- **Diet**: □Wet, □Dry; Brand/ Amt.:_____

Appetite	□Normal, □↑, □↓
Weight	□Normal, □↑, □↓; Past Wt.:_____ kg; Date:_____ ; Δ:_____
Thirst	□Normal, □↑, □↓
Urination	□Normal, □↑, □↓, □Blood, □Strain
Defecation	□Normal, □↑, □↓, □Blood, □Strain, □Diarrhea, □Mucus
Discharge	□No, □Yes; Onset/ Describe:
Cough/ Sneeze	□No, □Yes; Onset/ Describe:
Vomit	□No, □Yes; Onset/ Describe:
Respiration	□Normal, □↑ Rate, □↑ Effort
Energy level	□Normal, □Lethargic, □Exercise intolerance

- **Travel Hx**: □None, Other:_____
- **Exposure to**: □Standing water, □Wildlife, □Board/daycare, □Dog park, □Groomer
- **Adverse reactions to food/ meds**: □None, Other:_____
- **Can give oral meds**: □no □yes; Helpful Tricks:_____

Physical Exam:

T: P: R: Wt.:   BCS: Pain: CRT:

☐*CV*: Regular rhythm, no murmur, normokinetic and synchronous pulses
☐*Resp*: Normal BV sounds/ effort, normal tracheal sounds/ palpation
☐*Attitude*: Bright, alert, and responsive
☐*Hydration/ Perfusion*: MM pink and moist with a CRT of 1-2 sec
☐*Eyes*: No abnormalities
☐*Nose*: No abnormalities
☐*Ears*: No abnormalities; ☐Debris (mild / mod / sev) (AU / AD / AS)
☐*Oral cavity*: No abnormalities; ☐Tarter (mild / mod/ sev); ☐Gingivitis
☐*Lymph nodes*: Small, symmetrical, smooth, and soft
☐*Abdomen*: Soft, non-painful, no fluid-wave, organomegaly, or masses
☐*Mammary Chain*: No abnormalities
☐*Penis/ Vulva*: No abnormalities
☐*Skin*: No alopecia, masses, erythema, other lesions, or ectoparasites
☐*Neuro*: No paresis, ataxia, or postural deficits, normal PLR and mentation
☐*MS*: Adequate and symmetrical muscling, no overt lameness
☐*Rectal*: No abnormalities, normal colored feces on glove

Labwork:

Other Diagnostics:
Blood Pressure:

Problem List:

Plan:

Case No._____

Patient	Age	Sex	Breed	Weight
	DOB:	Mn / Mi Fs / Fi	Color:	kg

Owner	Primary Veterinarian	Admit Date/ Time
Name: Phone:	Name: Phone:	Date: Time: AM / PM

• **Presenting Complaint**:_____
_____
_____

• **Medical Hx**:_____
_____
_____

• **When/ where obtained**: Date:_____; ☐Breeder, ☐Shelter, Other:_____

Drug/ Suppl.	Amount	Dose (mg/kg)	Route	Frequency	Date Started

• **Vaccine status – Dog**: ☐Rab ☐Parv ☐Dist ☐Aden; ☐Para ☐Lep ☐Bord ☐Influ ☐Lyme
• **Vaccine status – Cat**: ☐Rab ☐Herp ☐Cali ☐Pan ☐FeLV[kittens]; ☐FIV ☐Chlam ☐Bord
• **Heartworm / Flea & Tick / Intestinal Parasites**:
  ○ *Last Heartworm Test*: Date:_____, ☐IDK; Test Results: ☐Pos, ☐Neg, ☐IDK
  ○ *Monthly heartworm preventative*: ☐no ☐yes, Product:_____
  ○ *Monthly flea & tick preventative*: ☐no ☐yes, Product:_____
  ○ *Monthly dewormer*: ☐no ☐yes, Product:_____
• **Surgical Hx**: ☐Spay/Neuter; Date:_____; Other:_____
• **Environment**: ☐Indoor, ☐Outdoor, Time spent outdoors/ Other:_____
• **Housemates**: Dogs:_____ Cats:_____ Other:_____
• **Diet**: ☐Wet, ☐Dry; Brand/ Amt.:_____

Appetite	☐Normal, ☐↑, ☐↓
Weight	☐Normal, ☐↑, ☐↓; Past Wt.:_____ kg; Date:_____; Δ:_____
Thirst	☐Normal, ☐↑, ☐↓
Urination	☐Normal, ☐↑, ☐↓, ☐Blood, ☐Strain
Defecation	☐Normal, ☐↑, ☐↓, ☐Blood, ☐Strain, ☐Diarrhea, ☐Mucus
Discharge	☐No, ☐Yes; Onset/ Describe:
Cough/ Sneeze	☐No, ☐Yes; Onset/ Describe:
Vomit	☐No, ☐Yes; Onset/ Describe:
Respiration	☐Normal, ☐↑ Rate, ☐↑ Effort
Energy level	☐Normal, ☐Lethargic, ☐Exercise intolerance

• **Travel Hx**: ☐None, Other:_____
• **Exposure to**: ☐Standing water, ☐Wildlife, ☐Board/daycare, ☐Dog park, ☐Groomer
• **Adverse reactions to food/ meds**: ☐None, Other:_____
• Can give oral meds: ☐no ☐yes; Helpful Tricks:_____

Physical Exam:

T: *P:*   *R:*   *Wt.:*   *BCS:*   *Pain:*   *CRT:*

☐*CV*: Regular rhythm, no murmur, normokinetic and synchronous pulses
☐*Resp*: Normal BV sounds/ effort, normal tracheal sounds/ palpation
☐*Attitude*: Bright, alert, and responsive
☐*Hydration/ Perfusion*: MM pink and moist with a CRT of 1-2 sec
☐*Eyes*: No abnormalities
☐*Nose*: No abnormalities
☐*Ears*: No abnormalities; ☐Debris (mild / mod / sev) (AU / AD / AS)
☐*Oral cavity*: No abnormalities; ☐Tarter (mild / mod/ sev); ☐Gingivitis
☐*Lymph nodes*: Small, symmetrical, smooth, and soft
☐*Abdomen*: Soft, non-painful, no fluid-wave, organomegaly, or masses
☐*Mammary Chain*: No abnormalities
☐*Penis/ Vulva*: No abnormalities
☐*Skin*: No alopecia, masses, erythema, other lesions, or ectoparasites
☐*Neuro*: No paresis, ataxia, or postural deficits, normal PLR and mentation
☐*MS*: Adequate and symmetrical muscling, no overt lameness
☐*Rectal*: No abnormalities, normal colored feces on glove

Labwork:

Other Diagnostics:
Blood Pressure:

Problem List:

Plan:

Case No._____

Patient	Age	Sex	Breed	Weight
	DOB:	Mn / Mi Fs / Fi	Color:	kg

Owner	Primary Veterinarian	Admit Date/ Time
Name: Phone:	Name: Phone:	Date: Time: AM / PM

- **Presenting Complaint**:_____
  _____
  _____

- **Medical Hx**:_____
  _____
  _____

- **When/ where obtained**: Date:_____; □Breeder, □Shelter, Other:_____

Drug/ Suppl.	Amount	Dose (mg/kg)	Route	Frequency	Date Started

- **Vaccine status – Dog**: □Rab □Parv □Dist □Aden; □Para □Lep □Bord □Influ □Lyme
- **Vaccine status – Cat**: □Rab □Herp □Cali □Pan □FeLV[kittens]; □FIV □Chlam □Bord
- **Heartworm / Flea & Tick / Intestinal Parasites**:
  - *Last Heartworm Test*: Date:_____, □IDK; Test Results: □Pos, □Neg, □IDK
  - *Monthly heartworm preventative*: □no □yes, Product:_____
  - *Monthly flea & tick preventative*: □no □yes, Product:_____
  - *Monthly dewormer*: □no □yes, Product:_____
- **Surgical Hx**: □Spay/Neuter; Date:_____; Other:_____
- **Environment**: □Indoor, □Outdoor, Time spent outdoors/ Other:_____
- **Housemates**: Dogs:_____ Cats:_____ Other:_____
- **Diet**: □Wet, □Dry; Brand/ Amt.:_____

Appetite	□Normal, □↑, □↓
Weight	□Normal, □↑, □↓; Past Wt.:_____ kg; Date:_____; Δ:_____
Thirst	□Normal, □↑, □↓
Urination	□Normal, □↑, □↓, □Blood, □Strain
Defecation	□Normal, □↑, □↓, □Blood, □Strain, □Diarrhea, □Mucus
Discharge	□No, □Yes; Onset/ Describe:
Cough/ Sneeze	□No, □Yes; Onset/ Describe:
Vomit	□No, □Yes; Onset/ Describe:
Respiration	□Normal, □↑ Rate, □↑ Effort
Energy level	□Normal, □Lethargic, □Exercise intolerance

- **Travel Hx**: □None, Other:_____
- **Exposure to**: □Standing water, □Wildlife, □Board/daycare, □Dog park, □Groomer
- **Adverse reactions to food/ meds**: □None, Other:_____
- **Can give oral meds**: □no □yes; Helpful Tricks:_____

Physical Exam:

T: *P*:   *R*:   *Wt.*:   *BCS*:   *Pain*:   *CRT*:

☐*CV*: Regular rhythm, no murmur, normokinetic and synchronous pulses
☐*Resp*: Normal BV sounds/ effort, normal tracheal sounds/ palpation
☐*Attitude*: Bright, alert, and responsive
☐*Hydration/ Perfusion*: MM pink and moist with a CRT of 1-2 sec
☐*Eyes*: No abnormalities
☐*Nose*: No abnormalities
☐*Ears*: No abnormalities; ☐Debris (mild / mod / sev) (AU / AD / AS)
☐*Oral cavity*: No abnormalities; ☐Tarter (mild / mod/ sev); ☐Gingivitis
☐*Lymph nodes*: Small, symmetrical, smooth, and soft
☐*Abdomen*: Soft, non-painful, no fluid-wave, organomegaly, or masses
☐*Mammary Chain*: No abnormalities
☐*Penis/ Vulva*: No abnormalities
☐*Skin*: No alopecia, masses, erythema, other lesions, or ectoparasites
☐*Neuro*: No paresis, ataxia, or postural deficits, normal PLR and mentation
☐*MS*: Adequate and symmetrical muscling, no overt lameness
☐*Rectal*: No abnormalities, normal colored feces on glove

Labwork:

Other Diagnostics:
Blood Pressure:

Problem List:

Plan:

Case No._____

Patient	Age	Sex	Breed	Weight
	DOB:	Mn / Mi Fs / Fi	Color:	kg

Owner	Primary Veterinarian	Admit Date/ Time
Name: Phone:	Name: Phone:	Date: Time: AM / PM

• **Presenting Complaint**:_____
_____
_____

• **Medical Hx**:_____
_____
_____

• **When/ where obtained**:   Date:_____; □Breeder, □Shelter, Other:_____

Drug/ Suppl.	Amount	Dose (mg/kg)	Route	Frequency	Date Started

• **Vaccine status – Dog**: □Rab □Parv □Dist □Aden; □Para □Lep □Bord □Influ □Lyme
• **Vaccine status – Cat**: □Rab □Herp □Cali □Pan □FeLV[kittens]; □FIV □Chlam □Bord
• **Heartworm / Flea & Tick / Intestinal Parasites**:
   ◦ *Last Heartworm Test*: Date:_____, □IDK; Test Results: □Pos, □Neg, □IDK
   ◦ *Monthly heartworm preventative*:   □no □yes, Product:_____
   ◦ *Monthly flea & tick preventative*: □no □yes, Product:_____
   ◦ *Monthly dewormer*:   □no □yes, Product:_____
• **Surgical Hx**:   □Spay/Neuter; Date:_____; Other:_____
• **Environment**: □Indoor, □Outdoor, Time spent outdoors/ Other:_____
• **Housemates**: Dogs:_____ Cats:_____ Other:_____
• **Diet**: □Wet, □Dry; Brand/ Amt.:_____

Appetite	□Normal, □↑, □↓
Weight	□Normal, □↑, □↓; Past Wt.:_____ kg; Date:_____; Δ:_____
Thirst	□Normal, □↑, □↓
Urination	□Normal, □↑, □↓, □Blood, □Strain
Defecation	□Normal, □↑, □↓, □Blood, □Strain, □Diarrhea, □Mucus
Discharge	□No, □Yes; Onset/ Describe:
Cough/ Sneeze	□No, □Yes; Onset/ Describe:
Vomit	□No, □Yes; Onset/ Describe:
Respiration	□Normal, □↑ Rate, □↑ Effort
Energy level	□Normal, □Lethargic, □Exercise intolerance

• **Travel Hx**: □None, Other:_____
• **Exposure to**: □Standing water, □Wildlife, □Board/daycare, □Dog park, □Groomer
• **Adverse reactions to food/ meds**: □None, Other:_____
• Can give oral meds: □no □yes; Helpful Tricks:_____

Physical Exam:

T: P: R: Wt.:   BCS: Pain: CRT:

☐*CV*: Regular rhythm, no murmur, normokinetic and synchronous pulses
☐*Resp*: Normal BV sounds/ effort, normal tracheal sounds/ palpation
☐*Attitude*: Bright, alert, and responsive
☐*Hydration/ Perfusion*: MM pink and moist with a CRT of 1-2 sec
☐*Eyes*: No abnormalities
☐*Nose*: No abnormalities
☐*Ears*: No abnormalities; ☐Debris (mild / mod / sev) (AU / AD / AS)
☐*Oral cavity*: No abnormalities; ☐Tarter (mild / mod/ sev); ☐Gingivitis
☐*Lymph nodes*: Small, symmetrical, smooth, and soft
☐*Abdomen*: Soft, non-painful, no fluid-wave, organomegaly, or masses
☐*Mammary Chain*: No abnormalities
☐*Penis/ Vulva*: No abnormalities
☐*Skin*: No alopecia, masses, erythema, other lesions, or ectoparasites
☐*Neuro*: No paresis, ataxia, or postural deficits, normal PLR and mentation
☐*MS*: Adequate and symmetrical muscling, no overt lameness
☐*Rectal*: No abnormalities, normal colored feces on glove

Labwork:

Other Diagnostics:
Blood Pressure:

Problem List:

Plan:

Patient	Age	Sex	Breed	Weight
	DOB:	Mn / Mi Fs / Fi	Color:	kg

Owner	Primary Veterinarian	Admit Date/ Time
Name: Phone:	Name: Phone:	Date: Time: AM / PM

• **Presenting Complaint**:_____
_____
_____

• **Medical Hx**:_____
_____
_____

• **When/ where obtained**: Date:_____; □Breeder, □Shelter, Other:_____

Drug/ Suppl.	Amount	Dose (mg/kg)	Route	Frequency	Date Started

• **Vaccine status – Dog**: □Rab □Parv □Dist □Aden; □Para □Lep □Bord □Influ □Lyme
• **Vaccine status – Cat**: □Rab □Herp □Cali □Pan □FeLV[kittens]; □FIV □Chlam □Bord
• **Heartworm / Flea & Tick / Intestinal Parasites**:
   ◦ *Last Heartworm Test*: Date:_____, □IDK; Test Results: □Pos, □Neg, □IDK
   ◦ *Monthly heartworm preventative*: □no □yes, Product:_____
   ◦ *Monthly flea & tick preventative*: □no □yes, Product:_____
   ◦ *Monthly dewormer*: □no □yes, Product:_____
• **Surgical Hx**: □Spay/Neuter; Date:_____; Other:_____
• **Environment**: □Indoor, □Outdoor, Time spent outdoors/ Other:_____
• **Housemates**: Dogs:_____ Cats:_____ Other:_____
• **Diet**: □Wet, □Dry; Brand/ Amt.:_____

Appetite	□Normal, □↑, □↓
Weight	□Normal, □↑, □↓; Past Wt.:_____kg; Date:_____; Δ:_____
Thirst	□Normal, □↑, □↓
Urination	□Normal, □↑, □↓, □Blood, □Strain
Defecation	□Normal, □↑, □↓, □Blood, □Strain, □Diarrhea, □Mucus
Discharge	□No, □Yes; Onset/ Describe:
Cough/ Sneeze	□No, □Yes; Onset/ Describe:
Vomit	□No, □Yes; Onset/ Describe:
Respiration	□Normal, □↑ Rate, □↑ Effort
Energy level	□Normal, □Lethargic, □Exercise intolerance

• **Travel Hx**: □None, Other:_____
• **Exposure to**: □Standing water, □Wildlife, □Board/daycare, □Dog park, □Groomer
• **Adverse reactions to food/ meds**: □None, Other:_____
• **Can give oral meds**: □no □yes; Helpful Tricks:_____

Physical Exam:

T: P: R: Wt.:   BCS: Pain: CRT:

☐*CV*: Regular rhythm, no murmur, normokinetic and synchronous pulses
☐*Resp*: Normal BV sounds/ effort, normal tracheal sounds/ palpation
☐*Attitude*: Bright, alert, and responsive
☐*Hydration/ Perfusion*: MM pink and moist with a CRT of 1-2 sec
☐*Eyes*: No abnormalities
☐*Nose*: No abnormalities
☐*Ears*: No abnormalities; ☐Debris (mild / mod / sev) (AU / AD / AS)
☐*Oral cavity*: No abnormalities; ☐Tarter (mild / mod/ sev); ☐Gingivitis
☐*Lymph nodes*: Small, symmetrical, smooth, and soft
☐*Abdomen*: Soft, non-painful, no fluid-wave, organomegaly, or masses
☐*Mammary Chain*: No abnormalities
☐*Penis/ Vulva*: No abnormalities
☐*Skin*: No alopecia, masses, erythema, other lesions, or ectoparasites
☐*Neuro*: No paresis, ataxia, or postural deficits, normal PLR and mentation
☐*MS*: Adequate and symmetrical muscling, no overt lameness
☐*Rectal*: No abnormalities, normal colored feces on glove

Labwork:

Other Diagnostics:
Blood Pressure:

Problem List:

Plan:

Case No._____

Patient	Age	Sex	Breed	Weight
	DOB:	Mn / Mi Fs / Fi	Color:	kg

Owner	Primary Veterinarian	Admit Date/ Time
Name: Phone:	Name: Phone:	Date: Time: AM / PM

• **Presenting Complaint**:_____

_____

• **Medical Hx**:_____

_____

• **When/ where obtained**:   Date:_____;   □Breeder, □Shelter, Other:_____

Drug/ Suppl.	Amount	Dose (mg/kg)	Route	Frequency	Date Started

• **Vaccine status – Dog**: □Rab □Parv □Dist □Aden; □Para □Lep □Bord □Influ □Lyme
• **Vaccine status – Cat**: □Rab □Herp □Cali □Pan □FeLV[kittens]; □FIV □Chlam □Bord
• **Heartworm / Flea & Tick / Intestinal Parasites**:
  ○ *Last Heartworm Test*: Date:_____, □IDK; Test Results: □Pos, □Neg, □IDK
  ○ *Monthly heartworm preventative*:   □no □yes, Product:_____
  ○ *Monthly flea & tick preventative*:   □no □yes, Product:_____
  ○ *Monthly dewormer*:   □no □yes, Product:_____
• **Surgical Hx**: □Spay/Neuter; Date:_____; Other:_____
• **Environment**: □Indoor, □Outdoor, Time spent outdoors/ Other:_____
• **Housemates**: Dogs:_____ Cats:_____ Other:_____
• **Diet**: □Wet, □Dry; Brand/ Amt.:_____

Appetite	□Normal, □↑, □↓
Weight	□Normal, □↑, □↓; Past Wt.:_____ kg; Date:_____; Δ:_____
Thirst	□Normal, □↑, □↓
Urination	□Normal, □↑, □↓, □Blood, □Strain
Defecation	□Normal, □↑, □↓, □Blood, □Strain, □Diarrhea, □Mucus
Discharge	□No, □Yes; Onset/ Describe:
Cough/ Sneeze	□No, □Yes; Onset/ Describe:
Vomit	□No, □Yes; Onset/ Describe:
Respiration	□Normal, □↑ Rate, □↑ Effort
Energy level	□Normal, □Lethargic, □Exercise intolerance

• **Travel Hx**: □None, Other:_____
• **Exposure to**: □Standing water, □Wildlife, □Board/daycare, □Dog park, □Groomer
• **Adverse reactions to food/ meds**: □None, Other:_____
• Can give oral meds: □no □yes; Helpful Tricks:_____

Physical Exam:

T: *P:*   *R:*   *Wt.:*   *BCS:*   *Pain:*   *CRT:*

☐*CV*: Regular rhythm, no murmur, normokinetic and synchronous pulses
☐*Resp*: Normal BV sounds/ effort, normal tracheal sounds/ palpation
☐*Attitude*: Bright, alert, and responsive
☐*Hydration/ Perfusion*: MM pink and moist with a CRT of 1-2 sec
☐*Eyes*: No abnormalities
☐*Nose*: No abnormalities
☐*Ears*: No abnormalities; ☐Debris (mild / mod / sev) (AU / AD / AS)
☐*Oral cavity*: No abnormalities; ☐Tarter (mild / mod/ sev); ☐Gingivitis
☐*Lymph nodes*: Small, symmetrical, smooth, and soft
☐*Abdomen*: Soft, non-painful, no fluid-wave, organomegaly, or masses
☐*Mammary Chain*: No abnormalities
☐*Penis/ Vulva*: No abnormalities
☐*Skin*: No alopecia, masses, erythema, other lesions, or ectoparasites
☐*Neuro*: No paresis, ataxia, or postural deficits, normal PLR and mentation
☐*MS*: Adequate and symmetrical muscling, no overt lameness
☐*Rectal*: No abnormalities, normal colored feces on glove

Labwork:

Other Diagnostics:
Blood Pressure:

Problem List:

Plan:

Case No._____

Patient	Age	Sex	Breed	Weight
	DOB:	Mn / Mi Fs / Fi	Color:	kg

Owner	Primary Veterinarian	Admit Date/ Time
Name: Phone:	Name: Phone:	Date: Time: AM / PM

• **Presenting Complaint**:_____
_____
_____

• **Medical Hx**:_____
_____
_____

• **When/ where obtained**:   Date:_____ ; □Breeder, □Shelter, Other:_____

Drug/ Suppl.	Amount	Dose (mg/kg)	Route	Frequency	Date Started

• **Vaccine status – Dog**: □Rab □Parv □Dist □Aden; □Para □Lep □Bord □Influ □Lyme
• **Vaccine status – Cat**: □Rab □Herp □Cali □Pan □FeLV[kittens]; □FIV □Chlam □Bord
• **Heartworm / Flea & Tick / Intestinal Parasites**:
  ◦ *Last Heartworm Test*: Date:_____, □IDK;   Test Results: □Pos, □Neg, □IDK
  ◦ *Monthly heartworm preventative*:   □no □yes,   Product:_____
  ◦ *Monthly flea & tick preventative*:   □no □yes,   Product:_____
  ◦ *Monthly dewormer*:   □no □yes,   Product:_____
• **Surgical Hx**:   □Spay/Neuter; Date:_____ ;   Other:_____
• **Environment**: □Indoor, □Outdoor, Time spent outdoors/ Other:_____
• **Housemates**: Dogs:_____ Cats:_____   Other:_____
• **Diet**: □Wet, □Dry; Brand/ Amt.:_____

Appetite	□Normal, □↑, □↓
Weight	□Normal, □↑, □↓; Past Wt.:_____ kg; Date:_____ ; Δ:_____
Thirst	□Normal, □↑, □↓
Urination	□Normal, □↑, □↓, □Blood, □Strain
Defecation	□Normal, □↑, □↓, □Blood, □Strain, □Diarrhea, □Mucus
Discharge	□No, □Yes; Onset/ Describe:
Cough/ Sneeze	□No, □Yes; Onset/ Describe:
Vomit	□No, □Yes; Onset/ Describe:
Respiration	□Normal, □↑ Rate, □↑ Effort
Energy level	□Normal, □Lethargic, □Exercise intolerance

• **Travel Hx**: □None, Other:_____
• **Exposure to**: □Standing water, □Wildlife, □Board/daycare, □Dog park, □Groomer
• **Adverse reactions to food/ meds**: □None, Other:_____
• Can give oral meds: □no □yes; Helpful Tricks:_____

Physical Exam:

T: P: R: Wt.:   BCS: Pain: CRT:

☐*CV*: Regular rhythm, no murmur, normokinetic and synchronous pulses
☐*Resp*: Normal BV sounds/ effort, normal tracheal sounds/ palpation
☐*Attitude*: Bright, alert, and responsive
☐*Hydration/ Perfusion*: MM pink and moist with a CRT of 1-2 sec
☐*Eyes*: No abnormalities
☐*Nose*: No abnormalities
☐*Ears*: No abnormalities; ☐Debris (mild / mod / sev) (AU / AD / AS)
☐*Oral cavity*: No abnormalities; ☐Tarter (mild / mod/ sev); ☐Gingivitis
☐*Lymph nodes*: Small, symmetrical, smooth, and soft
☐*Abdomen*: Soft, non-painful, no fluid-wave, organomegaly, or masses
☐*Mammary Chain*: No abnormalities
☐*Penis/ Vulva*: No abnormalities
☐*Skin*: No alopecia, masses, erythema, other lesions, or ectoparasites
☐*Neuro*: No paresis, ataxia, or postural deficits, normal PLR and mentation
☐*MS*: Adequate and symmetrical muscling, no overt lameness
☐*Rectal*: No abnormalities, normal colored feces on glove

Labwork:

Other Diagnostics:
Blood Pressure:

Problem List:

Plan:

Case No._____

Patient	Age	Sex	Breed	Weight
	DOB:	Mn / Mi Fs / Fi	Color:	kg

Owner	Primary Veterinarian	Admit Date/ Time
Name: Phone:	Name: Phone:	Date: Time: AM / PM

• **Presenting Complaint**:_____
_____
_____

• **Medical Hx**:_____
_____
_____

• **When/ where obtained**: Date:_____; ☐Breeder, ☐Shelter, Other:_____

Drug/ Suppl.	Amount	Dose (mg/kg)	Route	Frequency	Date Started

• **Vaccine status – Dog**: ☐Rab ☐Parv ☐Dist ☐Aden; ☐Para ☐Lep ☐Bord ☐Influ ☐Lyme
• **Vaccine status – Cat**: ☐Rab ☐Herp ☐Cali ☐Pan ☐FeLV[kittens]; ☐FIV ☐Chlam ☐Bord
• **Heartworm / Flea & Tick / Intestinal Parasites**:
  ◦ *Last Heartworm Test*: Date:_____, ☐IDK; Test Results: ☐Pos, ☐Neg, ☐IDK
  ◦ *Monthly heartworm preventative*: ☐no ☐yes, Product:_____
  ◦ *Monthly flea & tick preventative*: ☐no ☐yes, Product:_____
  ◦ *Monthly dewormer*: ☐no ☐yes, Product:_____
• **Surgical Hx**: ☐Spay/Neuter; Date:_____; Other:_____
• **Environment**: ☐Indoor, ☐Outdoor, Time spent outdoors/ Other:_____
• **Housemates**: Dogs:_____ Cats:_____ Other:_____
• **Diet**: ☐Wet, ☐Dry; Brand/ Amt.:_____

Appetite	☐Normal, ☐↑, ☐↓
Weight	☐Normal, ☐↑, ☐↓; Past Wt.:_____ kg; Date:_____; Δ:_____
Thirst	☐Normal, ☐↑, ☐↓
Urination	☐Normal, ☐↑, ☐↓, ☐Blood, ☐Strain
Defecation	☐Normal, ☐↑, ☐↓, ☐Blood, ☐Strain, ☐Diarrhea, ☐Mucus
Discharge	☐No, ☐Yes; Onset/ Describe:
Cough/ Sneeze	☐No, ☐Yes; Onset/ Describe:
Vomit	☐No, ☐Yes; Onset/ Describe:
Respiration	☐Normal, ☐↑ Rate, ☐↑ Effort
Energy level	☐Normal, ☐Lethargic, ☐Exercise intolerance

• **Travel Hx**: ☐None, Other:_____
• **Exposure to**: ☐Standing water, ☐Wildlife, ☐Board/daycare, ☐Dog park, ☐Groomer
• **Adverse reactions to food/ meds**: ☐None, Other:_____
• Can give oral meds: ☐no ☐yes; Helpful Tricks:_____

Physical Exam:

T: P: R: Wt.:   BCS: Pain: CRT:

☐*CV*: Regular rhythm, no murmur, normokinetic and synchronous pulses
☐*Resp*: Normal BV sounds/ effort, normal tracheal sounds/ palpation
☐*Attitude*: Bright, alert, and responsive
☐*Hydration/ Perfusion*: MM pink and moist with a CRT of 1-2 sec
☐*Eyes*: No abnormalities
☐*Nose*: No abnormalities
☐*Ears*: No abnormalities; ☐Debris (mild / mod / sev) (AU / AD / AS)
☐*Oral cavity*: No abnormalities; ☐Tarter (mild / mod/ sev); ☐Gingivitis
☐*Lymph nodes*: Small, symmetrical, smooth, and soft
☐*Abdomen*: Soft, non-painful, no fluid-wave, organomegaly, or masses
☐*Mammary Chain*: No abnormalities
☐*Penis/ Vulva*: No abnormalities
☐*Skin*: No alopecia, masses, erythema, other lesions, or ectoparasites
☐*Neuro*: No paresis, ataxia, or postural deficits, normal PLR and mentation
☐*MS*: Adequate and symmetrical muscling, no overt lameness
☐*Rectal*: No abnormalities, normal colored feces on glove

Labwork:

Other Diagnostics:
Blood Pressure:

Problem List:

Plan:

Patient		Age	Sex	Breed	Weight
	DOB:		Mn / Mi Fs / Fi	Color:	kg

Owner	Primary Veterinarian	Admit Date/ Time
Name: Phone:	Name: Phone:	Date: Time: AM / PM

• **Presenting Complaint**:_____
_____
_____
_____

• **Medical Hx**:_____
_____
_____

• **When/ where obtained**:   Date:_____; ☐Breeder, ☐Shelter, Other:_____

Drug/ Suppl.	Amount	Dose (mg/kg)	Route	Frequency	Date Started

• **Vaccine status – Dog**: ☐Rab ☐Parv ☐Dist ☐Aden; ☐Para ☐Lep ☐Bord ☐Influ ☐Lyme
• **Vaccine status – Cat**: ☐Rab ☐Herp ☐Cali ☐Pan ☐FeLV[kittens]; ☐FIV ☐Chlam ☐Bord
• **Heartworm / Flea & Tick / Intestinal Parasites**:
    ○ *Last Heartworm Test*: Date:_____, ☐IDK; Test Results: ☐Pos, ☐Neg, ☐IDK
    ○ *Monthly heartworm preventative*: ☐no ☐yes, Product:_____
    ○ *Monthly flea & tick preventative*: ☐no ☐yes, Product:_____
    ○ *Monthly dewormer*: ☐no ☐yes, Product:_____
• **Surgical Hx**: ☐Spay/Neuter; Date:_____; Other:_____
• **Environment**: ☐Indoor, ☐Outdoor, Time spent outdoors/ Other:_____
• **Housemates**: Dogs:_____ Cats:_____ Other:_____
• **Diet**: ☐Wet, ☐Dry; Brand/ Amt.:_____

Appetite	☐Normal, ☐↑, ☐↓
Weight	☐Normal, ☐↑, ☐↓; Past Wt.:_____ kg; Date:_____; Δ:_____
Thirst	☐Normal, ☐↑, ☐↓
Urination	☐Normal, ☐↑, ☐↓, ☐Blood, ☐Strain
Defecation	☐Normal, ☐↑, ☐↓, ☐Blood, ☐Strain, ☐Diarrhea, ☐Mucus
Discharge	☐No, ☐Yes; Onset/ Describe:
Cough/ Sneeze	☐No, ☐Yes; Onset/ Describe:
Vomit	☐No, ☐Yes; Onset/ Describe:
Respiration	☐Normal, ☐↑ Rate, ☐↑ Effort
Energy level	☐Normal, ☐Lethargic, ☐Exercise intolerance

• **Travel Hx**: ☐None, Other:_____
• **Exposure to**: ☐Standing water, ☐Wildlife, ☐Board/daycare, ☐Dog park, ☐Groomer
• **Adverse reactions to food/ meds**: ☐None, Other:_____
• Can give oral meds: ☐no ☐yes; Helpful Tricks:_____

Physical Exam:

T: *P:*   *R:*   *Wt.:*   *BCS:*   *Pain:*   *CRT:*

☐*CV*: Regular rhythm, no murmur, normokinetic and synchronous pulses
☐*Resp*: Normal BV sounds/ effort, normal tracheal sounds/ palpation
☐*Attitude*: Bright, alert, and responsive
☐*Hydration/ Perfusion*: MM pink and moist with a CRT of 1-2 sec
☐*Eyes*: No abnormalities
☐*Nose*: No abnormalities
☐*Ears*: No abnormalities; ☐Debris (mild / mod / sev) (AU / AD / AS)
☐*Oral cavity*: No abnormalities; ☐Tarter (mild / mod/ sev); ☐Gingivitis
☐*Lymph nodes*: Small, symmetrical, smooth, and soft
☐*Abdomen*: Soft, non-painful, no fluid-wave, organomegaly, or masses
☐*Mammary Chain*: No abnormalities
☐*Penis/ Vulva*: No abnormalities
☐*Skin*: No alopecia, masses, erythema, other lesions, or ectoparasites
☐*Neuro*: No paresis, ataxia, or postural deficits, normal PLR and mentation
☐*MS*: Adequate and symmetrical muscling, no overt lameness
☐*Rectal*: No abnormalities, normal colored feces on glove

Labwork:

Other Diagnostics:
Blood Pressure:

Problem List:

Plan:

Case No._____

Patient	Age	Sex	Breed	Weight
	DOB:	Mn / Mi Fs / Fi	Color:	kg

Owner	Primary Veterinarian	Admit Date/ Time
Name: Phone:	Name: Phone:	Date: Time: AM / PM

• **Presenting Complaint**:_____

_____

_____

• **Medical Hx**:_____

_____

_____

• **When/ where obtained**:   Date:_____; ☐Breeder, ☐Shelter, Other:_____

Drug/ Suppl.	Amount	Dose (mg/kg)	Route	Frequency	Date Started

• **Vaccine status – Dog**: ☐Rab ☐Parv ☐Dist ☐Aden; ☐Para ☐Lep ☐Bord ☐Influ ☐Lyme
• **Vaccine status – Cat**: ☐Rab ☐Herp ☐Cali ☐Pan ☐FeLV[kittens]; ☐FIV ☐Chlam ☐Bord
• **Heartworm / Flea & Tick / Intestinal Parasites**:
  ◦ *Last Heartworm Test*: Date:_____, ☐IDK; Test Results: ☐Pos, ☐Neg, ☐IDK
  ◦ *Monthly heartworm preventative*: ☐no ☐yes, Product:_____
  ◦ *Monthly flea & tick preventative*: ☐no ☐yes, Product:_____
  ◦ *Monthly dewormer*: ☐no ☐yes, Product:_____
• **Surgical Hx**:   ☐Spay/Neuter; Date:_____; Other:_____
• **Environment**: ☐Indoor, ☐Outdoor, Time spent outdoors/ Other:_____
• **Housemates**: Dogs:_____ Cats:_____ Other:_____
• **Diet**: ☐Wet, ☐Dry; Brand/ Amt.:_____

Appetite	☐Normal, ☐↑, ☐↓
Weight	☐Normal, ☐↑, ☐↓; Past Wt.:_____ kg; Date:_____; Δ:_____
Thirst	☐Normal, ☐↑, ☐↓
Urination	☐Normal, ☐↑, ☐↓, ☐Blood, ☐Strain
Defecation	☐Normal, ☐↑, ☐↓, ☐Blood, ☐Strain, ☐Diarrhea, ☐Mucus
Discharge	☐No, ☐Yes; Onset/ Describe:
Cough/ Sneeze	☐No, ☐Yes; Onset/ Describe:
Vomit	☐No, ☐Yes; Onset/ Describe:
Respiration	☐Normal, ☐↑ Rate, ☐↑ Effort
Energy level	☐Normal, ☐Lethargic, ☐Exercise intolerance

• **Travel Hx**: ☐None, Other:_____
• **Exposure to**: ☐Standing water, ☐Wildlife, ☐Board/daycare, ☐Dog park, ☐Groomer
• **Adverse reactions to food/ meds**: ☐None, Other:_____
• Can give oral meds: ☐no ☐yes; Helpful Tricks:_____

Physical Exam:

T: P: R: Wt.:   BCS: Pain: CRT:

☐*CV*: Regular rhythm, no murmur, normokinetic and synchronous pulses
☐*Resp*: Normal BV sounds/ effort, normal tracheal sounds/ palpation
☐*Attitude*: Bright, alert, and responsive
☐*Hydration/ Perfusion*: MM pink and moist with a CRT of 1-2 sec
☐*Eyes*: No abnormalities
☐*Nose*: No abnormalities
☐*Ears*: No abnormalities; ☐Debris (mild / mod / sev) (AU / AD / AS)
☐*Oral cavity*: No abnormalities; ☐Tarter (mild / mod/ sev); ☐Gingivitis
☐*Lymph nodes*: Small, symmetrical, smooth, and soft
☐*Abdomen*: Soft, non-painful, no fluid-wave, organomegaly, or masses
☐*Mammary Chain*: No abnormalities
☐*Penis/ Vulva*: No abnormalities
☐*Skin*: No alopecia, masses, erythema, other lesions, or ectoparasites
☐*Neuro*: No paresis, ataxia, or postural deficits, normal PLR and mentation
☐*MS*: Adequate and symmetrical muscling, no overt lameness
☐*Rectal*: No abnormalities, normal colored feces on glove

Labwork:

Other Diagnostics:
Blood Pressure:

Problem List:

Plan:

Case No._____

Patient	Age	Sex	Breed	Weight
	DOB:	Mn / Mi Fs / Fi	Color:	kg

Owner	Primary Veterinarian	Admit Date/ Time
Name: Phone:	Name: Phone:	Date: Time: AM / PM

• **Presenting Complaint**:_____
_____
_____

• **Medical Hx**:_____
_____
_____

• **When/ where obtained**: Date:_____; □Breeder, □Shelter, Other:_____

Drug/ Suppl.	Amount	Dose (mg/kg)	Route	Frequency	Date Started

• **Vaccine status – Dog**: □Rab □Parv □Dist □Aden; □Para □Lep □Bord □Influ □Lyme
• **Vaccine status – Cat**: □Rab □Herp □Cali □Pan □FeLV[kittens]; □FIV □Chlam □Bord
• **Heartworm / Flea & Tick / Intestinal Parasites**:
  ◦ *Last Heartworm Test*: Date:_____, □IDK; Test Results: □Pos, □Neg, □IDK
  ◦ *Monthly heartworm preventative*: □no □yes, Product:_____
  ◦ *Monthly flea & tick preventative*: □no □yes, Product:_____
  ◦ *Monthly dewormer*:   □no □yes, Product:_____
• **Surgical Hx**: □Spay/Neuter; Date:_____; Other:_____
• **Environment**: □Indoor, □Outdoor, Time spent outdoors/ Other:_____
• **Housemates**: Dogs:_____ Cats:_____ Other:_____
• **Diet**: □Wet, □Dry; Brand/ Amt.:_____

Appetite	□Normal, □↑, □↓
Weight	□Normal, □↑, □↓; Past Wt.:_____ kg; Date:_____; Δ:_____
Thirst	□Normal, □↑, □↓
Urination	□Normal, □↑, □↓, □Blood, □Strain
Defecation	□Normal, □↑, □↓, □Blood, □Strain, □Diarrhea, □Mucus
Discharge	□No, □Yes; Onset/ Describe:
Cough/ Sneeze	□No, □Yes; Onset/ Describe:
Vomit	□No, □Yes; Onset/ Describe:
Respiration	□Normal, □↑ Rate, □↑ Effort
Energy level	□Normal, □Lethargic, □Exercise intolerance

• **Travel Hx**: □None, Other:_____
• **Exposure to**: □Standing water, □Wildlife, □Board/daycare, □Dog park, □Groomer
• **Adverse reactions to food/ meds**: □None, Other:_____
• Can give oral meds: □no □yes; Helpful Tricks:_____

Physical Exam:

T: *P:*   *R:*   *Wt.:*   *BCS:*   *Pain:*   *CRT:*

☐*CV*: Regular rhythm, no murmur, normokinetic and synchronous pulses
☐*Resp*: Normal BV sounds/ effort, normal tracheal sounds/ palpation
☐*Attitude*: Bright, alert, and responsive
☐*Hydration/ Perfusion*: MM pink and moist with a CRT of 1-2 sec
☐*Eyes*: No abnormalities
☐*Nose*: No abnormalities
☐*Ears*: No abnormalities; ☐Debris (mild / mod / sev) (AU / AD / AS)
☐*Oral cavity*: No abnormalities; ☐Tarter (mild / mod/ sev); ☐Gingivitis
☐*Lymph nodes*: Small, symmetrical, smooth, and soft
☐*Abdomen*: Soft, non-painful, no fluid-wave, organomegaly, or masses
☐*Mammary Chain*: No abnormalities
☐*Penis/ Vulva*: No abnormalities
☐*Skin*: No alopecia, masses, erythema, other lesions, or ectoparasites
☐*Neuro*: No paresis, ataxia, or postural deficits, normal PLR and mentation
☐*MS*: Adequate and symmetrical muscling, no overt lameness
☐*Rectal*: No abnormalities, normal colored feces on glove

Labwork:

Other Diagnostics:
Blood Pressure:

Problem List:

Plan:

Case No._____

Patient	Age	Sex	Breed	Weight
	DOB:	Mn / Mi Fs / Fi	Color:	kg

Owner		Primary Veterinarian	Admit Date/ Time
Name: Phone:		Name: Phone:	Date: Time: AM / PM

• **Presenting Complaint**:_____

_____

• **Medical Hx**:_____

_____

• **When/ where obtained**: Date:_____; ☐Breeder, ☐Shelter, Other:_____

Drug/ Suppl.	Amount	Dose (mg/kg)	Route	Frequency	Date Started

• **Vaccine status – Dog**: ☐Rab ☐Parv ☐Dist ☐Aden; ☐Para ☐Lep ☐Bord ☐Influ ☐Lyme
• **Vaccine status – Cat**: ☐Rab ☐Herp ☐Cali ☐Pan ☐FeLV[kittens]; ☐FIV ☐Chlam ☐Bord
• **Heartworm / Flea & Tick / Intestinal Parasites**:
  ◦ *Last Heartworm Test*: Date:_____, ☐IDK; Test Results: ☐Pos, ☐Neg, ☐IDK
  ，◦ *Monthly heartworm preventative*: ☐no ☐yes, Product:_____
  ◦ *Monthly flea & tick preventative*: ☐no ☐yes, Product:_____
  ◦ *Monthly dewormer*:   ☐no ☐yes, Product:_____
• **Surgical Hx**: ☐Spay/Neuter; Date:_____; Other:_____
• **Environment**: ☐Indoor, ☐Outdoor, Time spent outdoors/ Other:_____
• **Housemates**: Dogs:_____ Cats:_____ Other:_____
• **Diet**: ☐Wet, ☐Dry; Brand/ Amt.:_____

Appetite	☐Normal, ☐↑, ☐↓
Weight	☐Normal, ☐↑, ☐↓; Past Wt.:_____ kg; Date:_____; Δ:_____
Thirst	☐Normal, ☐↑, ☐↓
Urination	☐Normal, ☐↑, ☐↓, ☐Blood, ☐Strain
Defecation	☐Normal, ☐↑, ☐↓, ☐Blood, ☐Strain, ☐Diarrhea, ☐Mucus
Discharge	☐No, ☐Yes; Onset/ Describe:
Cough/ Sneeze	☐No, ☐Yes; Onset/ Describe:
Vomit	☐No, ☐Yes; Onset/ Describe:
Respiration	☐Normal, ☐↑ Rate, ☐↑ Effort
Energy level	☐Normal, ☐Lethargic, ☐Exercise intolerance

• **Travel Hx**: ☐None, Other:_____
• **Exposure to**: ☐Standing water, ☐Wildlife, ☐Board/daycare, ☐Dog park, ☐Groomer
• **Adverse reactions to food/ meds**: ☐None, Other:_____
• Can give oral meds: ☐no ☐yes; Helpful Tricks:_____

Physical Exam:

T: P: R: Wt.:   BCS: Pain: CRT:

- ☐ *CV*: Regular rhythm, no murmur, normokinetic and synchronous pulses
- ☐ *Resp*: Normal BV sounds/ effort, normal tracheal sounds/ palpation
- ☐ *Attitude*: Bright, alert, and responsive
- ☐ *Hydration/ Perfusion*: MM pink and moist with a CRT of 1-2 sec
- ☐ *Eyes*: No abnormalities
- ☐ *Nose*: No abnormalities
- ☐ *Ears*: No abnormalities; ☐ Debris (mild / mod / sev) (AU / AD / AS)
- ☐ *Oral cavity*: No abnormalities; ☐ Tarter (mild / mod/ sev); ☐ Gingivitis
- ☐ *Lymph nodes*: Small, symmetrical, smooth, and soft
- ☐ *Abdomen*: Soft, non-painful, no fluid-wave, organomegaly, or masses
- ☐ *Mammary Chain*: No abnormalities
- ☐ *Penis/ Vulva*: No abnormalities
- ☐ *Skin*: No alopecia, masses, erythema, other lesions, or ectoparasites
- ☐ *Neuro*: No paresis, ataxia, or postural deficits, normal PLR and mentation
- ☐ *MS*: Adequate and symmetrical muscling, no overt lameness
- ☐ *Rectal*: No abnormalities, normal colored feces on glove

Labwork:

Other Diagnostics:
Blood Pressure:

Problem List:

Plan:

Case No._____

Patient	Age	Sex	Breed	Weight
	DOB:	Mn / Mi Fs / Fi	Color:	k

Owner	Primary Veterinarian	Admit Date/ Time
Name: Phone:	Name: Phone:	Date: Time: AM / PM

• **Presenting Complaint**:_____
_____
_____

• **Medical Hx**:_____
_____
_____

• **When/ where obtained**:   Date:_____; □Breeder, □Shelter, Other:_____

Drug/ Suppl.	Amount	Dose (mg/kg)	Route	Frequency	Date Started

• **Vaccine status – Dog**: □Rab □Parv □Dist □Aden; □Para □Lep □Bord □Influ □Lyme
• **Vaccine status – Cat**: □Rab □Herp □Cali □Pan □FeLV[kittens]; □FIV □Chlam □Bord
• **Heartworm / Flea & Tick / Intestinal Parasites**:
  ◦ *Last Heartworm Test*: Date:_____, □IDK; Test Results: □Pos, □Neg, □IDK
  ◦ *Monthly heartworm preventative*: □no □yes, Product:_____
  ◦ *Monthly flea & tick preventative*: □no □yes, Product:_____
  ◦ *Monthly dewormer*: □no □yes, Product:_____
• **Surgical Hx**:   □Spay/Neuter; Date:_____; Other:_____
• **Environment**: □Indoor, □Outdoor, Time spent outdoors/ Other:_____
• **Housemates**: Dogs:_____ Cats:_____ Other:_____
• **Diet**: □Wet, □Dry; Brand/ Amt.:_____

Appetite	□Normal, □↑, □↓
Weight	□Normal, □↑, □↓; Past Wt.:_____ kg; Date:_____; Δ:_____
Thirst	□Normal, □↑, □↓
Urination	□Normal, □↑, □↓, □Blood, □Strain
Defecation	□Normal, □↑, □↓, □Blood, □Strain, □Diarrhea, □Mucus
Discharge	□No, □Yes; Onset/ Describe:
Cough/ Sneeze	□No, □Yes; Onset/ Describe:
Vomit	□No, □Yes; Onset/ Describe:
Respiration	□Normal, □↑ Rate, □↑ Effort
Energy level	□Normal, □Lethargic, □Exercise intolerance

• **Travel Hx**: □None, Other:_____
• **Exposure to**: □Standing water, □Wildlife, □Board/daycare, □Dog park, □Groomer
• **Adverse reactions to food/ meds**: □None, Other:_____
• Can give oral meds: □no □yes; Helpful Tricks:_____

Physical Exam:

T: *P:*   *R:*   *Wt.:*   *BCS:*   *Pain:*   *CRT:*

☐*CV*: Regular rhythm, no murmur, normokinetic and synchronous pulses
☐*Resp*: Normal BV sounds/ effort, normal tracheal sounds/ palpation
☐*Attitude*: Bright, alert, and responsive
☐*Hydration/ Perfusion*: MM pink and moist with a CRT of 1-2 sec
☐*Eyes*: No abnormalities
☐*Nose*: No abnormalities
☐*Ears*: No abnormalities; ☐Debris (mild / mod / sev) (AU / AD / AS)
☐*Oral cavity*: No abnormalities; ☐Tarter (mild / mod/ sev); ☐Gingivitis
☐*Lymph nodes*: Small, symmetrical, smooth, and soft
☐*Abdomen*: Soft, non-painful, no fluid-wave, organomegaly, or masses
☐*Mammary Chain*: No abnormalities
☐*Penis/ Vulva*: No abnormalities
☐*Skin*: No alopecia, masses, erythema, other lesions, or ectoparasites
☐*Neuro*: No paresis, ataxia, or postural deficits, normal PLR and mentation
☐*MS*: Adequate and symmetrical muscling, no overt lameness
☐*Rectal*: No abnormalities, normal colored feces on glove

Labwork:

Other Diagnostics:
Blood Pressure:

Problem List:

Plan:

Patient	Age	Sex	Breed	Weight
	DOB:	Mn / Mi Fs / Fi	Color:	kg

Owner	Primary Veterinarian	Admit Date/ Time
Name: Phone:	Name: Phone:	Date: Time: AM / PM

• **Presenting Complaint**:_____
_____
_____

• **Medical Hx**:_____
_____
_____

• **When/ where obtained**: Date:_____; ☐Breeder, ☐Shelter, Other:_____

Drug/ Suppl.	Amount	Dose (mg/kg)	Route	Frequency	Date Started

• **Vaccine status – Dog**: ☐Rab ☐Parv ☐Dist ☐Aden; ☐Para ☐Lep ☐Bord ☐Influ ☐Lyme
• **Vaccine status – Cat**: ☐Rab ☐Herp ☐Cali ☐Pan ☐FeLV[kittens]; ☐FIV ☐Chlam ☐Bord
• **Heartworm / Flea & Tick / Intestinal Parasites**:
   ◦ *Last Heartworm Test*: Date:_____, ☐IDK; Test Results: ☐Pos, ☐Neg, ☐IDK
   ◦ *Monthly heartworm preventative*:   ☐no ☐yes, Product:_____
   ◦ *Monthly flea & tick preventative*:   ☐no ☐yes, Product:_____
   ◦ *Monthly dewormer*:   ☐no ☐yes, Product:_____
• **Surgical Hx**: ☐Spay/Neuter; Date:_____; Other:_____
• **Environment**: ☐Indoor, ☐Outdoor, Time spent outdoors/ Other:_____
• **Housemates**: Dogs:_____ Cats:_____ Other:_____
• **Diet**: ☐Wet, ☐Dry; Brand/ Amt.:_____

Appetite	☐Normal, ☐↑, ☐↓
Weight	☐Normal, ☐↑, ☐↓; Past Wt.:_____ kg; Date:_____; Δ:_____
Thirst	☐Normal, ☐↑, ☐↓
Urination	☐Normal, ☐↑, ☐↓, ☐Blood, ☐Strain
Defecation	☐Normal, ☐↑, ☐↓, ☐Blood, ☐Strain, ☐Diarrhea, ☐Mucus
Discharge	☐No, ☐Yes; Onset/ Describe:
Cough/ Sneeze	☐No, ☐Yes; Onset/ Describe:
Vomit	☐No, ☐Yes; Onset/ Describe:
Respiration	☐Normal, ☐↑ Rate, ☐↑ Effort
Energy level	☐Normal, ☐Lethargic, ☐Exercise intolerance

• **Travel Hx**: ☐None, Other:_____
• **Exposure to**: ☐Standing water, ☐Wildlife, ☐Board/daycare, ☐Dog park, ☐Groomer
• **Adverse reactions to food/ meds**: ☐None, Other:_____
• Can give oral meds: ☐no ☐yes; Helpful Tricks:_____

Physical Exam:

T: P: R: Wt.:   BCS: Pain: CRT:

☐*CV*: Regular rhythm, no murmur, normokinetic and synchronous pulses
☐*Resp*: Normal BV sounds/ effort, normal tracheal sounds/ palpation
☐*Attitude*: Bright, alert, and responsive
☐*Hydration/ Perfusion*: MM pink and moist with a CRT of 1-2 sec
☐*Eyes*: No abnormalities
☐*Nose*: No abnormalities
☐*Ears*: No abnormalities; ☐Debris (mild / mod / sev) (AU / AD / AS)
☐*Oral cavity*: No abnormalities; ☐Tarter (mild / mod/ sev); ☐Gingivitis
☐*Lymph nodes*: Small, symmetrical, smooth, and soft
☐*Abdomen*: Soft, non-painful, no fluid-wave, organomegaly, or masses
☐*Mammary Chain*: No abnormalities
☐*Penis/ Vulva*: No abnormalities
☐*Skin*: No alopecia, masses, erythema, other lesions, or ectoparasites
☐*Neuro*: No paresis, ataxia, or postural deficits, normal PLR and mentation
☐*MS*: Adequate and symmetrical muscling, no overt lameness
☐*Rectal*: No abnormalities, normal colored feces on glove

Labwork:

Other Diagnostics:
Blood Pressure:

Problem List:

Plan:

Case No._____

Patient	Age	Sex	Breed	Weight
	DOB:	Mn / Mi Fs / Fi	Color:	kg

Owner	Primary Veterinarian	Admit Date/ Time
Name: Phone:	Name: Phone:	Date: Time: AM / PM

• **Presenting Complaint**:_____

_____

• **Medical Hx**:_____

_____

• **When/ where obtained**: Date:_____; ☐Breeder, ☐Shelter, Other:_____

Drug/ Suppl.	Amount	Dose (mg/kg)	Route	Frequency	Date Started

• **Vaccine status – Dog**: ☐Rab ☐Parv ☐Dist ☐Aden; ☐Para ☐Lep ☐Bord ☐Influ ☐Lyme
• **Vaccine status – Cat**: ☐Rab ☐Herp ☐Cali ☐Pan ☐FeLV[kittens]; ☐FIV ☐Chlam ☐Bord
• **Heartworm / Flea & Tick / Intestinal Parasites**:
  ◦ *Last Heartworm Test*: Date:_____, ☐IDK; Test Results: ☐Pos, ☐Neg, ☐IDK
  ◦ *Monthly heartworm preventative*: ☐no ☐yes, Product:_____
  ◦ *Monthly flea & tick preventative*: ☐no ☐yes, Product:_____
  ◦ *Monthly dewormer*:   ☐no ☐yes, Product:_____
• **Surgical Hx**: ☐Spay/Neuter; Date:_____; Other:_____
• **Environment**: ☐Indoor, ☐Outdoor, Time spent outdoors/ Other:_____
• **Housemates**: Dogs:_____ Cats:_____ Other:_____
• **Diet**: ☐Wet, ☐Dry; Brand/ Amt.:_____

Appetite	☐Normal, ☐↑, ☐↓
Weight	☐Normal, ☐↑, ☐↓; Past Wt.:_____ kg; Date:_____; Δ:_____
Thirst	☐Normal, ☐↑, ☐↓
Urination	☐Normal, ☐↑, ☐↓, ☐Blood, ☐Strain
Defecation	☐Normal, ☐↑, ☐↓, ☐Blood, ☐Strain, ☐Diarrhea, ☐Mucus
Discharge	☐No, ☐Yes; Onset/ Describe:
Cough/ Sneeze	☐No, ☐Yes; Onset/ Describe:
Vomit	☐No, ☐Yes; Onset/ Describe:
Respiration	☐Normal, ☐↑ Rate, ☐↑ Effort
Energy level	☐Normal, ☐Lethargic, ☐Exercise intolerance

• **Travel Hx**: ☐None, Other:_____
• **Exposure to**: ☐Standing water, ☐Wildlife, ☐Board/daycare, ☐Dog park, ☐Groomer
• **Adverse reactions to food/ meds**: ☐None, Other:_____
• Can give oral meds: ☐no ☐yes; Helpful Tricks:_____

Physical Exam:

T: *P:*   *R:*   *Wt.:*   *BCS:*   *Pain:*   *CRT:*

☐*CV*: Regular rhythm, no murmur, normokinetic and synchronous pulses
☐*Resp*: Normal BV sounds/ effort, normal tracheal sounds/ palpation
☐*Attitude*: Bright, alert, and responsive
☐*Hydration/ Perfusion*: MM pink and moist with a CRT of 1-2 sec
☐*Eyes*: No abnormalities
☐*Nose*: No abnormalities
☐*Ears*: No abnormalities; ☐Debris (mild / mod / sev) (AU / AD / AS)
☐*Oral cavity*: No abnormalities; ☐Tarter (mild / mod/ sev); ☐Gingivitis
☐*Lymph nodes*: Small, symmetrical, smooth, and soft
☐*Abdomen*: Soft, non-painful, no fluid-wave, organomegaly, or masses
☐*Mammary Chain*: No abnormalities
☐*Penis/ Vulva*: No abnormalities
☐*Skin*: No alopecia, masses, erythema, other lesions, or ectoparasites
☐*Neuro*: No paresis, ataxia, or postural deficits, normal PLR and mentation
☐*MS*: Adequate and symmetrical muscling, no overt lameness
☐*Rectal*: No abnormalities, normal colored feces on glove

Labwork:

Other Diagnostics:
Blood Pressure:

Problem List:

Plan:

Case No._____

Patient	Age	Sex	Breed	Weight
	DOB:	Mn / Mi Fs / Fi	Color:	kg

Owner	Primary Veterinarian	Admit Date/ Time
Name: Phone:	Name: Phone:	Date: Time: AM / PM

• **Presenting Complaint**:_____
_____
_____

• **Medical Hx**:_____
_____
_____

• **When/ where obtained**:   Date:_____ ; □Breeder, □Shelter, Other:_____

Drug/ Suppl.	Amount	Dose (mg/kg)	Route	Frequency	Date Started

• **Vaccine status – Dog**: □Rab □Parv □Dist □Aden; □Para □Lep □Bord □Influ □Lyme
• **Vaccine status – Cat**: □Rab □Herp □Cali □Pan □FeLV[kittens]; □FIV □Chlam □Bord
• **Heartworm / Flea & Tick / Intestinal Parasites**:
  ◦ *Last Heartworm Test*: Date:_____, □IDK; Test Results: □Pos, □Neg, □IDK
  ◦ *Monthly heartworm preventative*: □no □yes, Product:_____
  ◦ *Monthly flea & tick preventative*: □no □yes, Product:_____
  ◦ *Monthly dewormer*:   □no □yes, Product:_____
• **Surgical Hx**:   □Spay/Neuter; Date:_____ ; Other:_____
• **Environment**: □Indoor, □Outdoor, Time spent outdoors/ Other:_____
• **Housemates**: Dogs:_____ Cats:_____ Other:_____
• **Diet**: □Wet, □Dry; Brand/ Amt.:_____

Appetite	□Normal, □↑, □↓
Weight	□Normal, □↑, □↓; Past Wt.:_____ kg; Date:_____ ; Δ:_____
Thirst	□Normal, □↑, □↓
Urination	□Normal, □↑, □↓, □Blood, □Strain
Defecation	□Normal, □↑, □↓, □Blood, □Strain, □Diarrhea, □Mucus
Discharge	□No, □Yes; Onset/ Describe:
Cough/ Sneeze	□No, □Yes; Onset/ Describe:
Vomit	□No, □Yes; Onset/ Describe:
Respiration	□Normal, □↑ Rate, □↑ Effort
Energy level	□Normal, □Lethargic, □Exercise intolerance

• **Travel Hx**: □None, Other:_____
• **Exposure to**: □Standing water, □Wildlife, □Board/daycare, □Dog park, □Groomer
• **Adverse reactions to food/ meds**: □None, Other:_____
• **Can give oral meds**: □no □yes; Helpful Tricks:_____

Physical Exam:

T: *P:*   *R:*   *Wt.:*   *BCS:*   *Pain:*   *CRT:*

☐*CV*: Regular rhythm, no murmur, normokinetic and synchronous pulses
☐*Resp*: Normal BV sounds/ effort, normal tracheal sounds/ palpation
☐*Attitude*: Bright, alert, and responsive
☐*Hydration/ Perfusion*: MM pink and moist with a CRT of 1-2 sec
☐*Eyes*: No abnormalities
☐*Nose*: No abnormalities
☐*Ears*: No abnormalities; ☐Debris (mild / mod / sev) (AU / AD / AS)
☐*Oral cavity*: No abnormalities; ☐Tarter (mild / mod/ sev); ☐Gingivitis
☐*Lymph nodes*: Small, symmetrical, smooth, and soft
☐*Abdomen*: Soft, non-painful, no fluid-wave, organomegaly, or masses
☐*Mammary Chain*: No abnormalities
☐*Penis/ Vulva*: No abnormalities
☐*Skin*: No alopecia, masses, erythema, other lesions, or ectoparasites
☐*Neuro*: No paresis, ataxia, or postural deficits, normal PLR and mentation
☐*MS*: Adequate and symmetrical muscling, no overt lameness
☐*Rectal*: No abnormalities, normal colored feces on glove

Labwork:

Other Diagnostics:
Blood Pressure:

Problem List:

Plan:

Case No._____

Patient	Age	Sex	Breed	Weight
	DOB:	Mn / Mi Fs / Fi	Color:	kg

Owner	Primary Veterinarian	Admit Date/ Time
Name: Phone:	Name: Phone:	Date: Time: AM / PM

• **Presenting Complaint**:_____
_____
_____

• **Medical Hx**:_____
_____
_____

• **When/ where obtained**:   Date:_____; ☐Breeder, ☐Shelter, Other:_____

Drug/ Suppl.	Amount	Dose (mg/kg)	Route	Frequency	Date Started

• **Vaccine status – Dog**: ☐Rab ☐Parv ☐Dist ☐Aden; ☐Para ☐Lep ☐Bord ☐Influ ☐Lyme
• **Vaccine status – Cat**: ☐Rab ☐Herp ☐Cali ☐Pan ☐FeLV[kittens]; ☐FIV ☐Chlam ☐Bord
• **Heartworm / Flea & Tick / Intestinal Parasites**:
   ◦ *Last Heartworm Test*: Date:_____, ☐IDK;   Test Results: ☐Pos, ☐Neg, ☐IDK
   ◦ *Monthly heartworm preventative*:   ☐no ☐yes,   Product:_____
   ◦ *Monthly flea & tick preventative*:   ☐no ☐yes,   Product:_____
   ◦ *Monthly dewormer*:   ☐no ☐yes,   Product:_____
• **Surgical Hx**:   ☐Spay/Neuter; Date:_____;   Other:_____
• **Environment**: ☐Indoor, ☐Outdoor, Time spent outdoors/ Other:_____
• **Housemates**: Dogs:_____ Cats:_____ Other:_____
• **Diet**: ☐Wet, ☐Dry; Brand/ Amt.:_____

Appetite	☐Normal, ☐↑, ☐↓
Weight	☐Normal, ☐↑, ☐↓; Past Wt.:_____ kg; Date:_____; Δ:_____
Thirst	☐Normal, ☐↑, ☐↓
Urination	☐Normal, ☐↑, ☐↓, ☐Blood, ☐Strain
Defecation	☐Normal, ☐↑, ☐↓, ☐Blood, ☐Strain, ☐Diarrhea, ☐Mucus
Discharge	☐No, ☐Yes; Onset/ Describe:
Cough/ Sneeze	☐No, ☐Yes; Onset/ Describe:
Vomit	☐No, ☐Yes; Onset/ Describe:
Respiration	☐Normal, ☐↑ Rate, ☐↑ Effort
Energy level	☐Normal, ☐Lethargic, ☐Exercise intolerance

• **Travel Hx**: ☐None, Other:_____
• **Exposure to**: ☐Standing water, ☐Wildlife, ☐Board/daycare, ☐Dog park, ☐Groomer
• **Adverse reactions to food/ meds**: ☐None, Other:_____
• **Can give oral meds**: ☐no ☐yes; Helpful Tricks:_____

Physical Exam:

T: P: R: Wt.:   BCS: Pain: CRT:

☐*CV*: Regular rhythm, no murmur, normokinetic and synchronous pulses
☐*Resp*: Normal BV sounds/ effort, normal tracheal sounds/ palpation
☐*Attitude*: Bright, alert, and responsive
☐*Hydration/ Perfusion*: MM pink and moist with a CRT of 1-2 sec
☐*Eyes*: No abnormalities
☐*Nose*: No abnormalities
☐*Ears*: No abnormalities; ☐Debris (mild / mod / sev) (AU / AD / AS)
☐*Oral cavity*: No abnormalities; ☐Tarter (mild / mod/ sev); ☐Gingivitis
☐*Lymph nodes*: Small, symmetrical, smooth, and soft
☐*Abdomen*: Soft, non-painful, no fluid-wave, organomegaly, or masses
☐*Mammary Chain*: No abnormalities
☐*Penis/ Vulva*: No abnormalities
☐*Skin*: No alopecia, masses, erythema, other lesions, or ectoparasites
☐*Neuro*: No paresis, ataxia, or postural deficits, normal PLR and mentation
☐*MS*: Adequate and symmetrical muscling, no overt lameness
☐*Rectal*: No abnormalities, normal colored feces on glove

Labwork:

Other Diagnostics:
Blood Pressure:

Problem List:

Plan:

Case No._____

Patient	Age	Sex	Breed	Weight
	DOB:	Mn / Mi Fs / Fi	Color:	kg

Owner	Primary Veterinarian	Admit Date/ Time
Name: Phone:	Name: Phone:	Date: Time: AM / PM

• **Presenting Complaint**:_____

_____

_____

• **Medical Hx**:_____

_____

_____

• **When/ where obtained**: Date:_____ ; □Breeder, □Shelter, Other:_____

Drug/ Suppl.	Amount	Dose (mg/kg)	Route	Frequency	Date Started

• **Vaccine status – Dog**: □Rab □Parv □Dist □Aden; □Para □Lep □Bord □Influ □Lyme
• **Vaccine status – Cat**: □Rab □Herp □Cali □Pan □FeLV[kittens]; □FIV □Chlam □Bord
• **Heartworm / Flea & Tick / Intestinal Parasites**:
  ∘ *Last Heartworm Test*: Date:_____, □IDK; Test Results: □Pos, □Neg, □IDK
  ∘ *Monthly heartworm preventative*: □no □yes, Product:_____
  ∘ *Monthly flea & tick preventative*: □no □yes, Product:_____
  ∘ *Monthly dewormer*: □no □yes, Product:_____
• **Surgical Hx**: □Spay/Neuter; Date:_____ ; Other:_____
• **Environment**: □Indoor, □Outdoor, Time spent outdoors/ Other:_____
• **Housemates**: Dogs:_____ Cats:_____ Other:_____
• **Diet**: □Wet, □Dry; Brand/ Amt.:_____

Appetite	□Normal, □↑, □↓
Weight	□Normal, □↑, □↓; Past Wt.:_____ kg; Date:_____ ; Δ:_____
Thirst	□Normal, □↑, □↓
Urination	□Normal, □↑, □↓, □Blood, □Strain
Defecation	□Normal, □↑, □↓, □Blood, □Strain, □Diarrhea, □Mucus
Discharge	□No, □Yes; Onset/ Describe:
Cough/ Sneeze	□No, □Yes; Onset/ Describe:
Vomit	□No, □Yes; Onset/ Describe:
Respiration	□Normal, □↑ Rate, □↑ Effort
Energy level	□Normal, □Lethargic, □Exercise intolerance

• **Travel Hx**: □None, Other:_____
• **Exposure to**: □Standing water, □Wildlife, □Board/daycare, □Dog park, □Groomer
• **Adverse reactions to food/ meds**: □None, Other:_____
• Can give oral meds: □no □yes; Helpful Tricks:_____

Physical Exam:

T: P: R: Wt.: BCS: Pain: CRT:

☐*CV*: Regular rhythm, no murmur, normokinetic and synchronous pulses
☐*Resp*: Normal BV sounds/ effort, normal tracheal sounds/ palpation
☐*Attitude*: Bright, alert, and responsive
☐*Hydration/ Perfusion*: MM pink and moist with a CRT of 1-2 sec
☐*Eyes*: No abnormalities
☐*Nose*: No abnormalities
☐*Ears*: No abnormalities; ☐Debris (mild / mod / sev) (AU / AD / AS)
☐*Oral cavity*: No abnormalities; ☐Tarter (mild / mod/ sev); ☐Gingivitis
☐*Lymph nodes*: Small, symmetrical, smooth, and soft
☐*Abdomen*: Soft, non-painful, no fluid-wave, organomegaly, or masses
☐*Mammary Chain*: No abnormalities
☐*Penis/ Vulva*: No abnormalities
☐*Skin*: No alopecia, masses, erythema, other lesions, or ectoparasites
☐*Neuro*: No paresis, ataxia, or postural deficits, normal PLR and mentation
☐*MS*: Adequate and symmetrical muscling, no overt lameness
☐*Rectal*: No abnormalities, normal colored feces on glove

Labwork:

Other Diagnostics:
Blood Pressure:

Problem List:

Plan:

Case No._____

Patient		Age	Sex	Breed	Weight
	DOB:		Mn / Mi Fs / Fi	Color:	kg

Owner	Primary Veterinarian	Admit Date/ Time
Name: Phone:	Name: Phone:	Date: Time: AM / PM

• **Presenting Complaint**:_____
_____
_____

• **Medical Hx**:_____
_____
_____

• **When/ where obtained**: Date:_____ ; □Breeder, □Shelter, Other:_____

Drug/ Suppl.	Amount	Dose (mg/kg)	Route	Frequency	Date Started

• **Vaccine status – Dog**: □Rab □Parv □Dist □Aden; □Para □Lep □Bord □Influ □Lyme
• **Vaccine status – Cat**: □Rab □Herp □Cali □Pan □FeLV[kittens]; □FIV □Chlam □Bord
• **Heartworm / Flea & Tick / Intestinal Parasites**:
  ○ *Last Heartworm Test*: Date:_____, □IDK; Test Results: □Pos, □Neg, □IDK
  ○ *Monthly heartworm preventative*: □no □yes, Product:_____
  ○ *Monthly flea & tick preventative*: □no □yes, Product:_____
  ○ *Monthly dewormer*: □no □yes, Product:_____
• **Surgical Hx**: □Spay/Neuter; Date:_____ ; Other:_____
• **Environment**: □Indoor, □Outdoor, Time spent outdoors/ Other:_____
• **Housemates**: Dogs:_____ Cats:_____ Other:_____
• **Diet**: □Wet, □Dry; Brand/ Amt.:_____

Appetite	□Normal, □↑, □↓
Weight	□Normal, □↑, □↓; Past Wt.:_____ kg; Date:_____ ; Δ:_____
Thirst	□Normal, □↑, □↓
Urination	□Normal, □↑, □↓, □Blood, □Strain
Defecation	□Normal, □↑, □↓, □Blood, □Strain, □Diarrhea, □Mucus
Discharge	□No, □Yes; Onset/ Describe:
Cough/ Sneeze	□No, □Yes; Onset/ Describe:
Vomit	□No, □Yes; Onset/ Describe:
Respiration	□Normal, □↑ Rate, □↑ Effort
Energy level	□Normal, □Lethargic, □Exercise intolerance

• **Travel Hx**: □None, Other:_____
• **Exposure to**: □Standing water, □Wildlife, □Board/daycare, □Dog park, □Groomer
• **Adverse reactions to food/ meds**: □None, Other:_____
• Can give oral meds: □no □yes; Helpful Tricks:_____

Physical Exam:

T: P: R: Wt.: BCS: Pain: CRT:

☐*CV*: Regular rhythm, no murmur, normokinetic and synchronous pulses
☐*Resp*: Normal BV sounds/ effort, normal tracheal sounds/ palpation
☐*Attitude*: Bright, alert, and responsive
☐*Hydration/ Perfusion*: MM pink and moist with a CRT of 1-2 sec
☐*Eyes*: No abnormalities
☐*Nose*: No abnormalities
☐*Ears*: No abnormalities; ☐Debris (mild / mod / sev) (AU / AD / AS)
☐*Oral cavity*: No abnormalities; ☐Tarter (mild / mod/ sev); ☐Gingivitis
☐*Lymph nodes*: Small, symmetrical, smooth, and soft
☐*Abdomen*: Soft, non-painful, no fluid-wave, organomegaly, or masses
☐*Mammary Chain*: No abnormalities
☐*Penis/ Vulva*: No abnormalities
☐*Skin*: No alopecia, masses, erythema, other lesions, or ectoparasites
☐*Neuro*: No paresis, ataxia, or postural deficits, normal PLR and mentation
☐*MS*: Adequate and symmetrical muscling, no overt lameness
☐*Rectal*: No abnormalities, normal colored feces on glove

Labwork:

Other Diagnostics:
Blood Pressure:

Problem List:

Plan:

Case No._____

Patient	Age	Sex	Breed	Weight
	DOB:	Mn / Mi Fs / Fi	Color:	kg

Owner		Primary Veterinarian	Admit Date/ Time
Name: Phone:		Name: Phone:	Date: Time: AM / PM

• **Presenting Complaint**:_____
_____
_____
_____

• **Medical Hx**:_____
_____
_____

• **When/ where obtained**:   Date:_____; □Breeder, □Shelter, Other:_____

Drug/ Suppl.	Amount	Dose (mg/kg)	Route	Frequency	Date Started

• **Vaccine status – Dog**: □Rab □Parv □Dist □Aden; □Para □Lep □Bord □Influ □Lyme
• **Vaccine status – Cat**: □Rab □Herp □Cali □Pan □FeLV[kittens]; □FIV □Chlam □Bord
• **Heartworm / Flea & Tick / Intestinal Parasites**:
   ◦ *Last Heartworm Test*: Date:_____, □IDK; Test Results: □Pos, □Neg, □IDK
   ◦ *Monthly heartworm preventative*:   □no □yes, Product:_____
   ◦ *Monthly flea & tick preventative*:   □no □yes, Product:_____
   ◦ *Monthly dewormer*:   □no □yes, Product:_____
• **Surgical Hx**:   □Spay/Neuter; Date:_____; Other:_____
• **Environment**: □Indoor, □Outdoor, Time spent outdoors/ Other:_____
• **Housemates**: Dogs:_____ Cats:_____ Other:_____
• **Diet**: □Wet, □Dry; Brand/ Amt.:_____

Appetite	□Normal, □↑, □↓
Weight	□Normal, □↑, □↓; Past Wt.:_____ kg; Date:_____; Δ:_____
Thirst	□Normal, □↑, □↓
Urination	□Normal, □↑, □↓, □Blood, □Strain
Defecation	□Normal, □↑, □↓, □Blood, □Strain, □Diarrhea, □Mucus
Discharge	□No, □Yes; Onset/ Describe:
Cough/ Sneeze	□No, □Yes; Onset/ Describe:
Vomit	□No, □Yes; Onset/ Describe:
Respiration	□Normal, □↑ Rate, □↑ Effort
Energy level	□Normal, □Lethargic, □Exercise intolerance

• **Travel Hx**: □None, Other:_____
• **Exposure to**: □Standing water, □Wildlife, □Board/daycare, □Dog park, □Groomer
• **Adverse reactions to food/ meds**: □None, Other:_____
• **Can give oral meds**: □no □yes; Helpful Tricks:_____

Physical Exam:

T: *P:*   *R:*   *Wt.:*   *BCS:*   *Pain:*   *CRT:*

☐*CV*: Regular rhythm, no murmur, normokinetic and synchronous pulses
☐*Resp*: Normal BV sounds/ effort, normal tracheal sounds/ palpation
☐*Attitude*: Bright, alert, and responsive
☐*Hydration/ Perfusion*: MM pink and moist with a CRT of 1-2 sec
☐*Eyes*: No abnormalities
☐*Nose*: No abnormalities
☐*Ears*: No abnormalities; ☐Debris (mild / mod / sev) (AU / AD / AS)
☐*Oral cavity*: No abnormalities; ☐Tarter (mild / mod/ sev); ☐Gingivitis
☐*Lymph nodes*: Small, symmetrical, smooth, and soft
☐*Abdomen*: Soft, non-painful, no fluid-wave, organomegaly, or masses
☐*Mammary Chain*: No abnormalities
☐*Penis/ Vulva*: No abnormalities
☐*Skin*: No alopecia, masses, erythema, other lesions, or ectoparasites
☐*Neuro*: No paresis, ataxia, or postural deficits, normal PLR and mentation
☐*MS*: Adequate and symmetrical muscling, no overt lameness
☐*Rectal*: No abnormalities, normal colored feces on glove

Labwork:

Other Diagnostics:
Blood Pressure:

Problem List:

Plan:

Case No._____

Patient	Age	Sex	Breed	Weight
	DOB:	Mn / Mi Fs / Fi	Color:	kg

Owner	Primary Veterinarian	Admit Date/ Time
Name: Phone:	Name: Phone:	Date: Time: AM / PM

• **Presenting Complaint**:_____
_____
_____

• **Medical Hx**:_____
_____
_____

• **When/ where obtained**: Date:_____; □Breeder, □Shelter, Other:_____

Drug/ Suppl.	Amount	Dose (mg/kg)	Route	Frequency	Date Started

• **Vaccine status – Dog**: □Rab □Parv □Dist □Aden; □Para □Lep □Bord □Influ □Lyme
• **Vaccine status – Cat**: □Rab □Herp □Cali □Pan □FeLV[kittens]; □FIV □Chlam □Bord
• **Heartworm / Flea & Tick / Intestinal Parasites**:
　○ *Last Heartworm Test*: Date:_____, □IDK; Test Results: □Pos, □Neg, □IDK
　○ *Monthly heartworm preventative*:　□no □yes, Product:_____
　○ *Monthly flea & tick preventative*:　□no □yes, Product:_____
　○ *Monthly dewormer*:　　　　　　　□no □yes, Product:_____
• **Surgical Hx**: □Spay/Neuter; Date:_____; Other:_____
• **Environment**: □Indoor, □Outdoor, Time spent outdoors/ Other:_____
• **Housemates**: Dogs:_____ Cats:_____ Other:_____
• **Diet**: □Wet, □Dry; Brand/ Amt.:_____

Appetite	□Normal, □↑, □↓
Weight	□Normal, □↑, □↓; Past Wt.:_____ kg; Date:_____; Δ:_____
Thirst	□Normal, □↑, □↓
Urination	□Normal, □↑, □↓, □Blood, □Strain
Defecation	□Normal, □↑, □↓, □Blood, □Strain, □Diarrhea, □Mucus
Discharge	□No, □Yes; Onset/ Describe:
Cough/ Sneeze	□No, □Yes; Onset/ Describe:
Vomit	□No, □Yes; Onset/ Describe:
Respiration	□Normal, □↑ Rate, □↑ Effort
Energy level	□Normal, □Lethargic, □Exercise intolerance

• **Travel Hx**: □None, Other:_____
• **Exposure to**: □Standing water, □Wildlife, □Board/daycare, □Dog park, □Groomer
• **Adverse reactions to food/ meds**: □None, Other:_____
• Can give oral meds: □no □yes; Helpful Tricks:_____

Physical Exam:

T:	P:	R:	Wt.:	BCS:	Pain:	CRT:

☐*CV*: Regular rhythm, no murmur, normokinetic and synchronous pulses
☐*Resp*: Normal BV sounds/ effort, normal tracheal sounds/ palpation
☐*Attitude*: Bright, alert, and responsive
☐*Hydration/ Perfusion*: MM pink and moist with a CRT of 1-2 sec
☐*Eyes*: No abnormalities
☐*Nose*: No abnormalities
☐*Ears*: No abnormalities; ☐Debris (mild / mod / sev) (AU / AD / AS)
☐*Oral cavity*: No abnormalities; ☐Tarter (mild / mod/ sev); ☐Gingivitis
☐*Lymph nodes*: Small, symmetrical, smooth, and soft
☐*Abdomen*: Soft, non-painful, no fluid-wave, organomegaly, or masses
☐*Mammary Chain*: No abnormalities
☐*Penis/ Vulva*: No abnormalities
☐*Skin*: No alopecia, masses, erythema, other lesions, or ectoparasites
☐*Neuro*: No paresis, ataxia, or postural deficits, normal PLR and mentation
☐*MS*: Adequate and symmetrical muscling, no overt lameness
☐*Rectal*: No abnormalities, normal colored feces on glove

Labwork:

Other Diagnostics:
Blood Pressure:

Problem List:

Plan:

Case No._____

Patient	Age	Sex	Breed	Weight
	DOB:	Mn / Mi Fs / Fi Color:		kg

Owner	Primary Veterinarian	Admit Date/ Time
Name: Phone:	Name: Phone:	Date: Time: AM / PM

• **Presenting Complaint**:_____
_____
_____

• **Medical Hx**:_____
_____
_____

• **When/ where obtained**:   Date:_____; □Breeder, □Shelter, Other:_____

Drug/ Suppl.	Amount	Dose (mg/kg)	Route	Frequency	Date Started

• **Vaccine status – Dog**: □Rab □Parv □Dist □Aden; □Para □Lep □Bord □Influ □Lyme
• **Vaccine status – Cat**: □Rab □Herp □Cali □Pan □FeLV[kittens]; □FIV □Chlam □Bord
• **Heartworm / Flea & Tick / Intestinal Parasites**:
  ○ *Last Heartworm Test*: Date:_____, □IDK; Test Results: □Pos, □Neg, □IDK
  ○ *Monthly heartworm preventative*: □no □yes, Product:_____
  ○ *Monthly flea & tick preventative*: □no □yes, Product:_____
  ○ *Monthly dewormer*:   □no □yes, Product:_____
• **Surgical Hx**: □Spay/Neuter; Date:_____; Other:_____
• **Environment**: □Indoor, □Outdoor, Time spent outdoors/ Other:_____
• **Housemates**: Dogs:_____ Cats:_____ Other:_____
• **Diet**: □Wet, □Dry; Brand/ Amt.:_____

Appetite	□Normal, □↑, □↓
Weight	□Normal, □↑, □↓; Past Wt.:_____ kg; Date:_____; Δ:_____
Thirst	□Normal, □↑, □↓
Urination	□Normal, □↑, □↓, □Blood, □Strain
Defecation	□Normal, □↑, □↓, □Blood, □Strain, □Diarrhea, □Mucus
Discharge	□No, □Yes; Onset/ Describe:
Cough/ Sneeze	□No, □Yes; Onset/ Describe:
Vomit	□No, □Yes; Onset/ Describe:
Respiration	□Normal, □↑ Rate, □↑ Effort
Energy level	□Normal, □Lethargic, □Exercise intolerance

• **Travel Hx**: □None, Other:_____
• **Exposure to**: □Standing water, □Wildlife, □Board/daycare, □Dog park, □Groomer
• **Adverse reactions to food/ meds**: □None, Other:_____
• **Can give oral meds**: □no □yes; Helpful Tricks:_____

Physical Exam:

T: P: R: Wt.:   BCS: Pain: CRT:

☐*CV*: Regular rhythm, no murmur, normokinetic and synchronous pulses
☐*Resp*: Normal BV sounds/ effort, normal tracheal sounds/ palpation
☐*Attitude*: Bright, alert, and responsive
☐*Hydration/ Perfusion*: MM pink and moist with a CRT of 1-2 sec
☐*Eyes*: No abnormalities
☐*Nose*: No abnormalities
☐*Ears*: No abnormalities; ☐Debris (mild / mod / sev) (AU / AD / AS)
☐*Oral cavity*: No abnormalities; ☐Tarter (mild / mod/ sev); ☐Gingivitis
☐*Lymph nodes*: Small, symmetrical, smooth, and soft
☐*Abdomen*: Soft, non-painful, no fluid-wave, organomegaly, or masses
☐*Mammary Chain*: No abnormalities
☐*Penis/ Vulva*: No abnormalities
☐*Skin*: No alopecia, masses, erythema, other lesions, or ectoparasites
☐*Neuro*: No paresis, ataxia, or postural deficits, normal PLR and mentation
☐*MS*: Adequate and symmetrical muscling, no overt lameness
☐*Rectal*: No abnormalities, normal colored feces on glove

Labwork:

Other Diagnostics:
Blood Pressure:

Problem List:

Plan:

Case No._____

Patient	Age	Sex	Breed	Weight
	DOB:	Mn / Mi Fs / Fi	Color:	kg

Owner		Primary Veterinarian	Admit Date/ Time
Name: Phone:		Name: Phone:	Date: Time: AM / PM

• **Presenting Complaint**:_____

_____

_____

• **Medical Hx**:_____

_____

_____

• **When/ where obtained**:   Date:_____; ☐Breeder, ☐Shelter, Other:_____

Drug/ Suppl.	Amount	Dose (mg/kg)	Route	Frequency	Date Started

• **Vaccine status – Dog**: ☐Rab ☐Parv ☐Dist ☐Aden; ☐Para ☐Lep ☐Bord ☐Influ ☐Lyme
• **Vaccine status – Cat**: ☐Rab ☐Herp ☐Cali ☐Pan ☐FeLV[kittens]; ☐FIV ☐Chlam ☐Bord
• **Heartworm / Flea & Tick / Intestinal Parasites**:
   ○ *Last Heartworm Test*: Date:_____, ☐IDK;   Test Results: ☐Pos, ☐Neg, ☐IDK
   ○ *Monthly heartworm preventative*:   ☐no ☐yes,   Product:_____
   ○ *Monthly flea & tick preventative*:   ☐no ☐yes,   Product:_____
   ○ *Monthly dewormer*:   ☐no ☐yes,   Product:_____
• **Surgical Hx**:   ☐Spay/Neuter; Date:_____;   Other:_____
• **Environment**: ☐Indoor, ☐Outdoor, Time spent outdoors/ Other:_____
• **Housemates**: Dogs:_____ Cats:_____ Other:_____
• **Diet**: ☐Wet, ☐Dry; Brand/ Amt.:_____

Appetite	☐Normal, ☐↑, ☐↓
Weight	☐Normal, ☐↑, ☐↓; Past Wt.:_____ kg; Date:_____; Δ:_____
Thirst	☐Normal, ☐↑, ☐↓
Urination	☐Normal, ☐↑, ☐↓, ☐Blood, ☐Strain
Defecation	☐Normal, ☐↑, ☐↓, ☐Blood, ☐Strain, ☐Diarrhea, ☐Mucus
Discharge	☐No, ☐Yes; Onset/ Describe:
Cough/ Sneeze	☐No, ☐Yes; Onset/ Describe:
Vomit	☐No, ☐Yes; Onset/ Describe:
Respiration	☐Normal, ☐↑ Rate, ☐↑ Effort
Energy level	☐Normal, ☐Lethargic, ☐Exercise intolerance

• **Travel Hx**: ☐None, Other:_____
• **Exposure to**: ☐Standing water, ☐Wildlife, ☐Board/daycare, ☐Dog park, ☐Groomer
• **Adverse reactions to food/ meds**: ☐None, Other:_____
• Can give oral meds: ☐no ☐yes; Helpful Tricks:_____

Physical Exam:

T: P: R: Wt.:   BCS: Pain: CRT:

☐*CV*: Regular rhythm, no murmur, normokinetic and synchronous pulses
☐*Resp*: Normal BV sounds/ effort, normal tracheal sounds/ palpation
☐*Attitude*: Bright, alert, and responsive
☐*Hydration/ Perfusion*: MM pink and moist with a CRT of 1-2 sec
☐*Eyes*: No abnormalities
☐*Nose*: No abnormalities
☐*Ears*: No abnormalities; ☐Debris (mild / mod / sev) (AU / AD / AS)
☐*Oral cavity*: No abnormalities; ☐Tarter (mild / mod/ sev); ☐Gingivitis
☐*Lymph nodes*: Small, symmetrical, smooth, and soft
☐*Abdomen*: Soft, non-painful, no fluid-wave, organomegaly, or masses
☐*Mammary Chain*: No abnormalities
☐*Penis/ Vulva*: No abnormalities
☐*Skin*: No alopecia, masses, erythema, other lesions, or ectoparasites
☐*Neuro*: No paresis, ataxia, or postural deficits, normal PLR and mentation
☐*MS*: Adequate and symmetrical muscling, no overt lameness
☐*Rectal*: No abnormalities, normal colored feces on glove

Labwork:

Other Diagnostics:
Blood Pressure:

Problem List:

Plan:

Case No._____

Patient	Age	Sex	Breed	Weight
	DOB:	Mn / Mi Fs / Fi	Color:	kg

Owner		Primary Veterinarian	Admit Date/ Time
Name: Phone:		Name: Phone:	Date: Time: AM / PM

• **Presenting Complaint**:_____

_____

_____

• **Medical Hx**:_____

_____

_____

• **When/ where obtained**:   Date:_____; □Breeder, □Shelter, Other:_____

Drug/ Suppl.	Amount	Dose (mg/kg)	Route	Frequency	Date Started

• **Vaccine status – Dog**: □Rab □Parv □Dist □Aden; □Para □Lep □Bord □Influ □Lyme
• **Vaccine status – Cat**: □Rab □Herp □Cali □Pan □FeLV[kittens]; □FIV □Chlam □Bord
• **Heartworm / Flea & Tick / Intestinal Parasites**:
  ◦ *Last Heartworm Test*: Date:_____, □IDK; Test Results: □Pos, □Neg, □IDK
  ◦ *Monthly heartworm preventative*:   □no □yes,   Product:_____
  ◦ *Monthly flea & tick preventative*:   □no □yes,   Product:_____
  ◦ *Monthly dewormer*:   □no □yes,   Product:_____
• **Surgical Hx**:   □Spay/Neuter; Date:_____; Other:_____
• **Environment**: □Indoor, □Outdoor, Time spent outdoors/ Other:_____
• **Housemates**: Dogs:_____ Cats:_____ Other:_____
• **Diet**: □Wet, □Dry; Brand/ Amt.:_____

Appetite	□Normal, □↑, □↓
Weight	□Normal, □↑, □↓; Past Wt.:_____ kg; Date:_____; Δ:_____
Thirst	□Normal, □↑, □↓
Urination	□Normal, □↑, □↓, □Blood, □Strain
Defecation	□Normal, □↑, □↓, □Blood, □Strain, □Diarrhea, □Mucus
Discharge	□No, □Yes; Onset/ Describe:
Cough/ Sneeze	□No, □Yes; Onset/ Describe:
Vomit	□No, □Yes; Onset/ Describe:
Respiration	□Normal, □↑ Rate, □↑ Effort
Energy level	□Normal, □Lethargic, □Exercise intolerance

• **Travel Hx**: □None, Other:_____
• **Exposure to**: □Standing water, □Wildlife, □Board/daycare, □Dog park, □Groomer
• **Adverse reactions to food/ meds**: □None, Other:_____
• Can give oral meds: □no □yes; Helpful Tricks:_____

Physical Exam:

T: *P:* *R:* *Wt.:* *BCS:* *Pain:* *CRT:*

☐*CV*: Regular rhythm, no murmur, normokinetic and synchronous pulses
☐*Resp*: Normal BV sounds/ effort, normal tracheal sounds/ palpation
☐*Attitude*: Bright, alert, and responsive
☐*Hydration/ Perfusion*: MM pink and moist with a CRT of 1-2 sec
☐*Eyes*: No abnormalities
☐*Nose*: No abnormalities
☐*Ears*: No abnormalities; ☐Debris (mild / mod / sev) (AU / AD / AS)
☐*Oral cavity*: No abnormalities; ☐Tarter (mild / mod/ sev); ☐Gingivitis
☐*Lymph nodes*: Small, symmetrical, smooth, and soft
☐*Abdomen*: Soft, non-painful, no fluid-wave, organomegaly, or masses
☐*Mammary Chain*: No abnormalities
☐*Penis/ Vulva*: No abnormalities
☐*Skin*: No alopecia, masses, erythema, other lesions, or ectoparasites
☐*Neuro*: No paresis, ataxia, or postural deficits, normal PLR and mentation
☐*MS*: Adequate and symmetrical muscling, no overt lameness
☐*Rectal*: No abnormalities, normal colored feces on glove

Labwork:

Other Diagnostics:
Blood Pressure:

Problem List:

Plan:

157

Patient	Age	Sex	Breed	Weight
	DOB:	Mn / Mi Fs / Fi Color:		kg

Owner	Primary Veterinarian	Admit Date/ Time
Name: Phone:	Name: Phone:	Date: Time: AM / PM

• **Presenting Complaint**:_____
_____
_____

• **Medical Hx**:_____
_____
_____

• **When/ where obtained**: Date:_____; ☐Breeder, ☐Shelter, Other:_____

Drug/ Suppl.	Amount	Dose (mg/kg)	Route	Frequency	Date Started

• **Vaccine status – Dog**: ☐Rab ☐Parv ☐Dist ☐Aden; ☐Para ☐Lep ☐Bord ☐Influ ☐Lyme
• **Vaccine status – Cat**: ☐Rab ☐Herp ☐Cali ☐Pan ☐FeLV[kittens]; ☐FIV ☐Chlam ☐Bord
• **Heartworm / Flea & Tick / Intestinal Parasites**:
   ◦ *Last Heartworm Test*: Date:_____, ☐IDK; Test Results: ☐Pos, ☐Neg, ☐IDK
   ◦ *Monthly heartworm preventative*: ☐no ☐yes, Product:_____
   ◦ *Monthly flea & tick preventative*: ☐no ☐yes, Product:_____
   ◦ *Monthly dewormer*: ☐no ☐yes, Product:_____
• **Surgical Hx**: ☐Spay/Neuter; Date:_____; Other:_____
• **Environment**: ☐Indoor, ☐Outdoor, Time spent outdoors/ Other:_____
• **Housemates**: Dogs:_____ Cats:_____ Other:_____
• **Diet**: ☐Wet, ☐Dry; Brand/ Amt.:_____

Appetite	☐Normal, ☐↑, ☐↓
Weight	☐Normal, ☐↑, ☐↓; Past Wt.:_____ kg; Date:_____; Δ:_____
Thirst	☐Normal, ☐↑, ☐↓
Urination	☐Normal, ☐↑, ☐↓, ☐Blood, ☐Strain
Defecation	☐Normal, ☐↑, ☐↓, ☐Blood, ☐Strain, ☐Diarrhea, ☐Mucus
Discharge	☐No, ☐Yes; Onset/ Describe:
Cough/ Sneeze	☐No, ☐Yes; Onset/ Describe:
Vomit	☐No, ☐Yes; Onset/ Describe:
Respiration	☐Normal, ☐↑ Rate, ☐↑ Effort
Energy level	☐Normal, ☐Lethargic, ☐Exercise intolerance

• **Travel Hx**: ☐None, Other:_____
• **Exposure to**: ☐Standing water, ☐Wildlife, ☐Board/daycare, ☐Dog park, ☐Groomer
• **Adverse reactions to food/ meds**: ☐None, Other:_____
• **Can give oral meds**: ☐no ☐yes; Helpful Tricks:_____

Physical Exam:

T: P: R: Wt.:   BCS: Pain: CRT:

☐*CV*: Regular rhythm, no murmur, normokinetic and synchronous pulses
☐*Resp*: Normal BV sounds/ effort, normal tracheal sounds/ palpation
☐*Attitude*: Bright, alert, and responsive
☐*Hydration/ Perfusion*: MM pink and moist with a CRT of 1-2 sec
☐*Eyes*: No abnormalities
☐*Nose*: No abnormalities
☐*Ears*: No abnormalities; ☐Debris (mild / mod / sev) (AU / AD / AS)
☐*Oral cavity*: No abnormalities; ☐Tarter (mild / mod/ sev); ☐Gingivitis
☐*Lymph nodes*: Small, symmetrical, smooth, and soft
☐*Abdomen*: Soft, non-painful, no fluid-wave, organomegaly, or masses
☐*Mammary Chain*: No abnormalities
☐*Penis/ Vulva*: No abnormalities
☐*Skin*: No alopecia, masses, erythema, other lesions, or ectoparasites
☐*Neuro*: No paresis, ataxia, or postural deficits, normal PLR and mentation
☐*MS*: Adequate and symmetrical muscling, no overt lameness
☐*Rectal*: No abnormalities, normal colored feces on glove

Labwork:

Other Diagnostics:
Blood Pressure:

Problem List:

Plan:

Case No._____

Patient	Age	Sex	Breed	Weight
	DOB:	Mn / Mi Fs / Fi	Color:	kg

Owner		Primary Veterinarian	Admit Date/ Time
Name: Phone:		Name: Phone:	Date: Time: AM / PM

• **Presenting Complaint**:_____
_____
_____

• **Medical Hx**:_____
_____
_____

• **When/ where obtained**: Date:_____; ☐Breeder, ☐Shelter, Other:_____

Drug/ Suppl.	Amount	Dose (mg/kg)	Route	Frequency	Date Started

• **Vaccine status – Dog**: ☐Rab ☐Parv ☐Dist ☐Aden; ☐Para ☐Lep ☐Bord ☐Influ ☐Lyme
• **Vaccine status – Cat**: ☐Rab ☐Herp ☐Cali ☐Pan ☐FeLV[kittens]; ☐FIV ☐Chlam ☐Bord
• **Heartworm / Flea & Tick / Intestinal Parasites**:
  ◦ *Last Heartworm Test*: Date:_____, ☐IDK; Test Results: ☐Pos, ☐Neg, ☐IDK
  ◦ *Monthly heartworm preventative*: ☐no ☐yes, Product:_____
  ◦ *Monthly flea & tick preventative*: ☐no ☐yes, Product:_____
  ◦ *Monthly dewormer*: ☐no ☐yes, Product:_____
• **Surgical Hx**: ☐Spay/Neuter; Date:_____; Other:_____
• **Environment**: ☐Indoor, ☐Outdoor, Time spent outdoors/ Other:_____
• **Housemates**: Dogs:_____ Cats:_____ Other:_____
• **Diet**: ☐Wet, ☐Dry; Brand/ Amt.:_____

Appetite	☐Normal, ☐↑, ☐↓
Weight	☐Normal, ☐↑, ☐↓; Past Wt.:_____ kg; Date:_____; Δ:_____
Thirst	☐Normal, ☐↑, ☐↓
Urination	☐Normal, ☐↑, ☐↓, ☐Blood, ☐Strain
Defecation	☐Normal, ☐↑, ☐↓, ☐Blood, ☐Strain, ☐Diarrhea, ☐Mucus
Discharge	☐No, ☐Yes; Onset/ Describe:
Cough/ Sneeze	☐No, ☐Yes; Onset/ Describe:
Vomit	☐No, ☐Yes; Onset/ Describe:
Respiration	☐Normal, ☐↑ Rate, ☐↑ Effort
Energy level	☐Normal, ☐Lethargic, ☐Exercise intolerance

• **Travel Hx**: ☐None, Other:_____
• **Exposure to**: ☐Standing water, ☐Wildlife, ☐Board/daycare, ☐Dog park, ☐Groomer
• **Adverse reactions to food/ meds**: ☐None, Other:_____
• Can give oral meds: ☐no ☐yes; Helpful Tricks:_____

Physical Exam:

T: *P:*   *R:*   *Wt.:*   *BCS:*   *Pain:*   *CRT:*

☐*CV*: Regular rhythm, no murmur, normokinetic and synchronous pulses
☐*Resp*: Normal BV sounds/ effort, normal tracheal sounds/ palpation
☐*Attitude*: Bright, alert, and responsive
☐*Hydration/ Perfusion*: MM pink and moist with a CRT of 1-2 sec
☐*Eyes*: No abnormalities
☐*Nose*: No abnormalities
☐*Ears*: No abnormalities; ☐Debris (mild / mod / sev) (AU / AD / AS)
☐*Oral cavity*: No abnormalities; ☐Tarter (mild / mod/ sev); ☐Gingivitis
☐*Lymph nodes*: Small, symmetrical, smooth, and soft
☐*Abdomen*: Soft, non-painful, no fluid-wave, organomegaly, or masses
☐*Mammary Chain*: No abnormalities
☐*Penis/ Vulva*: No abnormalities
☐*Skin*: No alopecia, masses, erythema, other lesions, or ectoparasites
☐*Neuro*: No paresis, ataxia, or postural deficits, normal PLR and mentation
☐*MS*: Adequate and symmetrical muscling, no overt lameness
☐*Rectal*: No abnormalities, normal colored feces on glove

Labwork:

Other Diagnostics:
Blood Pressure:

Problem List:

Plan:

Case No._____

Patient	Age	Sex	Breed	Weight
	DOB:	Mn / Mi Fs / Fi	Color:	kg

Owner	Primary Veterinarian	Admit Date/ Time
Name: Phone:	Name: Phone:	Date: Time: AM / PM

• **Presenting Complaint**:_____

_____

• **Medical Hx**:_____

_____

• **When/ where obtained**: Date:_____; ☐Breeder, ☐Shelter, Other:_____

Drug/ Suppl.	Amount	Dose (mg/kg)	Route	Frequency	Date Started

• **Vaccine status – Dog**: ☐Rab ☐Parv ☐Dist ☐Aden; ☐Para ☐Lep ☐Bord ☐Influ ☐Lyme
• **Vaccine status – Cat**: ☐Rab ☐Herp ☐Cali ☐Pan ☐FeLV[kittens]; ☐FIV ☐Chlam ☐Bord
• **Heartworm / Flea & Tick / Intestinal Parasites**:
  ◦ *Last Heartworm Test*: Date:_____, ☐IDK; Test Results: ☐Pos, ☐Neg, ☐IDK
  ◦ *Monthly heartworm preventative*: ☐no ☐yes, Product:_____
  ◦ *Monthly flea & tick preventative*: ☐no ☐yes, Product:_____
  ◦ *Monthly dewormer*: ☐no ☐yes, Product:_____
• **Surgical Hx**: ☐Spay/Neuter; Date:_____; Other:_____
• **Environment**: ☐Indoor, ☐Outdoor, Time spent outdoors/ Other:_____
• **Housemates**: Dogs:_____ Cats:_____ Other:_____
• **Diet**: ☐Wet, ☐Dry; Brand/ Amt.:_____

Appetite	☐Normal, ☐↑, ☐↓
Weight	☐Normal, ☐↑, ☐↓; Past Wt.:_____ kg; Date:_____; Δ:_____
Thirst	☐Normal, ☐↑, ☐↓
Urination	☐Normal, ☐↑, ☐↓, ☐Blood, ☐Strain
Defecation	☐Normal, ☐↑, ☐↓, ☐Blood, ☐Strain, ☐Diarrhea, ☐Mucus
Discharge	☐No, ☐Yes; Onset/ Describe:
Cough/ Sneeze	☐No, ☐Yes; Onset/ Describe:
Vomit	☐No, ☐Yes; Onset/ Describe:
Respiration	☐Normal, ☐↑ Rate, ☐↑ Effort
Energy level	☐Normal, ☐Lethargic, ☐Exercise intolerance

• **Travel Hx**: ☐None, Other:_____
• **Exposure to**: ☐Standing water, ☐Wildlife, ☐Board/daycare, ☐Dog park, ☐Groomer
• **Adverse reactions to food/ meds**: ☐None, Other:_____
• Can give oral meds: ☐no ☐yes; Helpful Tricks:_____

Physical Exam:

T: *P*:   *R*:   *Wt.*:   *BCS*:   *Pain*:   *CRT*:

☐*CV*: Regular rhythm, no murmur, normokinetic and synchronous pulses
☐*Resp*: Normal BV sounds/ effort, normal tracheal sounds/ palpation
☐*Attitude*: Bright, alert, and responsive
☐*Hydration/ Perfusion*: MM pink and moist with a CRT of 1-2 sec
☐*Eyes*: No abnormalities
☐*Nose*: No abnormalities
☐*Ears*: No abnormalities;   ☐Debris (mild / mod / sev) (AU / AD / AS)
☐*Oral cavity*: No abnormalities;   ☐Tarter (mild / mod/ sev);   ☐Gingivitis
☐*Lymph nodes*: Small, symmetrical, smooth, and soft
☐*Abdomen*: Soft, non-painful, no fluid-wave, organomegaly, or masses
☐*Mammary Chain*: No abnormalities
☐*Penis/ Vulva*: No abnormalities
☐*Skin*: No alopecia, masses, erythema, other lesions, or ectoparasites
☐*Neuro*: No paresis, ataxia, or postural deficits, normal PLR and mentation
☐*MS*: Adequate and symmetrical muscling, no overt lameness
☐*Rectal*: No abnormalities, normal colored feces on glove

Labwork:

Other Diagnostics:
Blood Pressure:

Problem List:

Plan:

Patient	Age	Sex	Breed	Weight
	DOB:	Mn / Mi Fs / Fi	Color:	kg

Owner	Primary Veterinarian	Admit Date/ Time
Name: Phone:	Name: Phone:	Date: Time: AM / PM

• **Presenting Complaint**:_____
_____
_____

• **Medical Hx**:_____
_____
_____

• **When/ where obtained**:   Date:_____; ☐Breeder, ☐Shelter, Other:_____

Drug/ Suppl.	Amount	Dose (mg/kg)	Route	Frequency	Date Started

• **Vaccine status – Dog**: ☐Rab ☐Parv ☐Dist ☐Aden; ☐Para ☐Lep ☐Bord ☐Influ ☐Lyme
• **Vaccine status – Cat**: ☐Rab ☐Herp ☐Cali ☐Pan ☐FeLV[kittens]; ☐FIV ☐Chlam ☐Bord
• **Heartworm / Flea & Tick / Intestinal Parasites**:
  ◦ *Last Heartworm Test*: Date:_____, ☐IDK; Test Results: ☐Pos, ☐Neg, ☐IDK
  ◦ *Monthly heartworm preventative*: ☐no ☐yes, Product:_____
  ◦ *Monthly flea & tick preventative*: ☐no ☐yes, Product:_____
  ◦ *Monthly dewormer*:   ☐no ☐yes, Product:_____
• **Surgical Hx**: ☐Spay/Neuter; Date:_____; Other:_____
• **Environment**: ☐Indoor, ☐Outdoor, Time spent outdoors/ Other:_____
• **Housemates**: Dogs:_____ Cats:_____ Other:_____
• **Diet**: ☐Wet, ☐Dry; Brand/ Amt.:_____

Appetite	☐Normal, ☐↑, ☐↓
Weight	☐Normal, ☐↑, ☐↓; Past Wt.:_____ kg; Date:_____; Δ:_____
Thirst	☐Normal, ☐↑, ☐↓
Urination	☐Normal, ☐↑, ☐↓, ☐Blood, ☐Strain
Defecation	☐Normal, ☐↑, ☐↓, ☐Blood, ☐Strain, ☐Diarrhea, ☐Mucus
Discharge	☐No, ☐Yes; Onset/ Describe:
Cough/ Sneeze	☐No, ☐Yes; Onset/ Describe:
Vomit	☐No, ☐Yes; Onset/ Describe:
Respiration	☐Normal, ☐↑ Rate, ☐↑ Effort
Energy level	☐Normal, ☐Lethargic, ☐Exercise intolerance

• **Travel Hx**: ☐None, Other:_____
• **Exposure to**: ☐Standing water, ☐Wildlife, ☐Board/daycare, ☐Dog park, ☐Groomer
• **Adverse reactions to food/ meds**: ☐None, Other:_____
• Can give oral meds: ☐no ☐yes; Helpful Tricks:_____

Physical Exam:

T: *P:*   *R:*   *Wt.:*   *BCS:*   *Pain:*   *CRT:*

☐*CV*: Regular rhythm, no murmur, normokinetic and synchronous pulses
☐*Resp*: Normal BV sounds/ effort, normal tracheal sounds/ palpation
☐*Attitude*: Bright, alert, and responsive
☐*Hydration/ Perfusion*: MM pink and moist with a CRT of 1-2 sec
☐*Eyes*: No abnormalities
☐*Nose*: No abnormalities
☐*Ears*: No abnormalities; ☐Debris (mild / mod / sev) (AU / AD / AS)
☐*Oral cavity*: No abnormalities; ☐Tarter (mild / mod/ sev); ☐Gingivitis
☐*Lymph nodes*: Small, symmetrical, smooth, and soft
☐*Abdomen*: Soft, non-painful, no fluid-wave, organomegaly, or masses
☐*Mammary Chain*: No abnormalities
☐*Penis/ Vulva*: No abnormalities
☐*Skin*: No alopecia, masses, erythema, other lesions, or ectoparasites
☐*Neuro*: No paresis, ataxia, or postural deficits, normal PLR and mentation
☐*MS*: Adequate and symmetrical muscling, no overt lameness
☐*Rectal*: No abnormalities, normal colored feces on glove

Labwork:

Other Diagnostics:
Blood Pressure:

Problem List:

Plan:

Case No._____

Patient	Age	Sex	Breed	Weight
	DOB:	Mn / Mi Fs / Fi	Color:	kg

Owner	Primary Veterinarian	Admit Date/ Time
Name: Phone:	Name: Phone:	Date: Time: AM / PM

• **Presenting Complaint**:_____
_____
_____

• **Medical Hx**:_____
_____
_____

• **When/ where obtained**: Date:_____; □Breeder, □Shelter, Other:_____

Drug/ Suppl.	Amount	Dose (mg/kg)	Route	Frequency	Date Started

• **Vaccine status – Dog**: □Rab □Parv □Dist □Aden; □Para □Lep □Bord □Influ □Lyme
• **Vaccine status – Cat**: □Rab □Herp □Cali □Pan □FeLV[kittens]; □FIV □Chlam □Bord
• **Heartworm / Flea & Tick / Intestinal Parasites**:
  ◦ *Last Heartworm Test*: Date:_____, □IDK; Test Results: □Pos, □Neg, □IDK
  ◦ *Monthly heartworm preventative*: □no □yes, Product:_____
  ◦ *Monthly flea & tick preventative*: □no □yes, Product:_____
  ◦ *Monthly dewormer*: □no □yes, Product:_____
• **Surgical Hx**: □Spay/Neuter; Date:_____; Other:_____
• **Environment**: □Indoor, □Outdoor, Time spent outdoors/ Other:_____
• **Housemates**: Dogs:_____ Cats:_____ Other:_____
• **Diet**: □Wet, □Dry; Brand/ Amt.:_____

Appetite	□Normal, □↑, □↓
Weight	□Normal, □↑, □↓; Past Wt.:_____ kg; Date:_____; Δ:_____
Thirst	□Normal, □↑, □↓
Urination	□Normal, □↑, □↓, □Blood, □Strain
Defecation	□Normal, □↑, □↓, □Blood, □Strain, □Diarrhea, □Mucus
Discharge	□No, □Yes; Onset/ Describe:
Cough/ Sneeze	□No, □Yes; Onset/ Describe:
Vomit	□No, □Yes; Onset/ Describe:
Respiration	□Normal, □↑ Rate, □↑ Effort
Energy level	□Normal, □Lethargic, □Exercise intolerance

• **Travel Hx**: □None, Other:_____
• **Exposure to**: □Standing water, □Wildlife, □Board/daycare, □Dog park, □Groomer
• **Adverse reactions to food/ meds**: □None, Other:_____
• Can give oral meds: □no □yes; Helpful Tricks:_____

Physical Exam:

T:　　　　*P:*　　　　*R:*　　　　*Wt.:*　　　　*BCS:*　　　*Pain:*　　　*CRT:*

☐*CV*: Regular rhythm, no murmur, normokinetic and synchronous pulses
☐*Resp*: Normal BV sounds/ effort, normal tracheal sounds/ palpation
☐*Attitude*: Bright, alert, and responsive
☐*Hydration/ Perfusion*: MM pink and moist with a CRT of 1-2 sec
☐*Eyes*: No abnormalities
☐*Nose*: No abnormalities
☐*Ears*: No abnormalities; ☐Debris (mild / mod / sev) (AU / AD / AS)
☐*Oral cavity*: No abnormalities; ☐Tarter (mild / mod/ sev); ☐Gingivitis
☐*Lymph nodes*: Small, symmetrical, smooth, and soft
☐*Abdomen*: Soft, non-painful, no fluid-wave, organomegaly, or masses
☐*Mammary Chain*: No abnormalities
☐*Penis/ Vulva*: No abnormalities
☐*Skin*: No alopecia, masses, erythema, other lesions, or ectoparasites
☐*Neuro*: No paresis, ataxia, or postural deficits, normal PLR and mentation
☐*MS*: Adequate and symmetrical muscling, no overt lameness
☐*Rectal*: No abnormalities, normal colored feces on glove

Labwork:

Other Diagnostics:
Blood Pressure:

Problem List:

Plan:

Case No._____

Patient	Age	Sex	Breed	Weight
	DOB:	Mn / Mi Fs / Fi	Color:	kg

Owner		Primary Veterinarian	Admit Date/ Time
Name: Phone:		Name: Phone:	Date: Time: AM / PM

• **Presenting Complaint**:_____
_____
_____

• **Medical Hx**:_____
_____
_____

• **When/ where obtained**:   Date:_____; □Breeder, □Shelter, Other:_____

Drug/ Suppl.	Amount	Dose (mg/kg)	Route	Frequency	Date Started

• **Vaccine status – Dog**: □Rab □Parv □Dist □Aden; □Para □Lep □Bord □Influ □Lyme
• **Vaccine status – Cat**: □Rab □Herp □Cali □Pan □FeLV[kittens]; □FIV □Chlam □Bord
• **Heartworm / Flea & Tick / Intestinal Parasites**:
   ◦ *Last Heartworm Test*: Date:_____, □IDK; Test Results: □Pos, □Neg, □IDK
   ◦ *Monthly heartworm preventative*: □no □yes, Product:_____
   ◦ *Monthly flea & tick preventative*: □no □yes, Product:_____
   ◦ *Monthly dewormer*:   □no □yes, Product:_____
• **Surgical Hx**:   □Spay/Neuter; Date:_____; Other:_____
• **Environment**: □Indoor, □Outdoor, Time spent outdoors/ Other:_____
• **Housemates**: Dogs:_____ Cats:_____ Other:_____
• **Diet**: □Wet, □Dry; Brand/ Amt.:_____

Appetite	□Normal, □↑, □↓
Weight	□Normal, □↑, □↓; Past Wt.:_____ kg; Date:_____; Δ:_____
Thirst	□Normal, □↑, □↓
Urination	□Normal, □↑, □↓, □Blood, □Strain
Defecation	□Normal, □↑, □↓, □Blood, □Strain, □Diarrhea, □Mucus
Discharge	□No, □Yes; Onset/ Describe:
Cough/ Sneeze	□No, □Yes; Onset/ Describe:
Vomit	□No, □Yes; Onset/ Describe:
Respiration	□Normal, □↑ Rate, □↑ Effort
Energy level	□Normal, □Lethargic, □Exercise intolerance

• **Travel Hx**: □None, Other:_____
• **Exposure to**: □Standing water, □Wildlife, □Board/daycare, □Dog park, □Groomer
• **Adverse reactions to food/ meds**: □None, Other:_____
• Can give oral meds: □no □yes; Helpful Tricks:_____

Physical Exam:

T: P: R: Wt.:   BCS: Pain: CRT:

☐*CV*: Regular rhythm, no murmur, normokinetic and synchronous pulses
☐*Resp*: Normal BV sounds/ effort, normal tracheal sounds/ palpation
☐*Attitude*: Bright, alert, and responsive
☐*Hydration/ Perfusion*: MM pink and moist with a CRT of 1-2 sec
☐*Eyes*: No abnormalities
☐*Nose*: No abnormalities
☐*Ears*: No abnormalities;   ☐Debris (mild / mod / sev) (AU / AD / AS)
☐*Oral cavity*: No abnormalities;   ☐Tarter (mild / mod/ sev);   ☐Gingivitis
☐*Lymph nodes*: Small, symmetrical, smooth, and soft
☐*Abdomen*: Soft, non-painful, no fluid-wave, organomegaly, or masses
☐*Mammary Chain*: No abnormalities
☐*Penis/ Vulva*: No abnormalities
☐*Skin*: No alopecia, masses, erythema, other lesions, or ectoparasites
☐*Neuro*: No paresis, ataxia, or postural deficits, normal PLR and mentation
☐*MS*: Adequate and symmetrical muscling, no overt lameness
☐*Rectal*: No abnormalities, normal colored feces on glove

Labwork:

Other Diagnostics:
Blood Pressure:

Problem List:

Plan:

Patient	Age	Sex	Breed	Weight
	DOB:	Mn / Mi Fs / Fi	Color:	kg

Owner		Primary Veterinarian	Admit Date/ Time
Name: Phone:		Name: Phone:	Date: Time: AM / PM

• **Presenting Complaint**:_____

• **Medical Hx**:_____

• **When/ where obtained**:   Date:_____ ; ☐Breeder, ☐Shelter, Other:_____

Drug/ Suppl.	Amount	Dose (mg/kg)	Route	Frequency	Date Started

• **Vaccine status – Dog**: ☐Rab ☐Parv ☐Dist ☐Aden; ☐Para ☐Lep ☐Bord ☐Influ ☐Lyme
• **Vaccine status – Cat**: ☐Rab ☐Herp ☐Cali ☐Pan ☐FeLV[kittens]; ☐FIV ☐Chlam ☐Bord
• **Heartworm / Flea & Tick / Intestinal Parasites**:
   ○ *Last Heartworm Test*: Date:_____, ☐IDK; Test Results: ☐Pos, ☐Neg, ☐IDK
   ○ *Monthly heartworm preventative*:   ☐no ☐yes,   Product:_____
   ○ *Monthly flea & tick preventative*:   ☐no ☐yes,   Product:_____
   ○ *Monthly dewormer*:   ☐no ☐yes,   Product:_____
• **Surgical Hx**:   ☐Spay/Neuter; Date:_____;   Other:_____
• **Environment**: ☐Indoor, ☐Outdoor, Time spent outdoors/ Other:_____
• **Housemates**: Dogs:_____ Cats:_____ Other:_____
• **Diet**: ☐Wet, ☐Dry; Brand/ Amt.:_____

Appetite	☐Normal, ☐↑, ☐↓
Weight	☐Normal, ☐↑, ☐↓; Past Wt.:_____ kg; Date:_____; Δ:_____
Thirst	☐Normal, ☐↑, ☐↓
Urination	☐Normal, ☐↑, ☐↓, ☐Blood, ☐Strain
Defecation	☐Normal, ☐↑, ☐↓, ☐Blood, ☐Strain, ☐Diarrhea, ☐Mucus
Discharge	☐No, ☐Yes; Onset/ Describe:
Cough/ Sneeze	☐No, ☐Yes; Onset/ Describe:
Vomit	☐No, ☐Yes; Onset/ Describe:
Respiration	☐Normal, ☐↑ Rate, ☐↑ Effort
Energy level	☐Normal, ☐Lethargic, ☐Exercise intolerance

• **Travel Hx**: ☐None, Other:_____
• **Exposure to**: ☐Standing water, ☐Wildlife, ☐Board/daycare, ☐Dog park, ☐Groomer
• **Adverse reactions to food/ meds**: ☐None, Other:_____
• Can give oral meds: ☐no ☐yes; Helpful Tricks:_____

Physical Exam:

T: *P:*   *R:*   *Wt.:*   *BCS:*   *Pain:*   *CRT:*

☐*CV*: Regular rhythm, no murmur, normokinetic and synchronous pulses
☐*Resp*: Normal BV sounds/ effort, normal tracheal sounds/ palpation
☐*Attitude*: Bright, alert, and responsive
☐*Hydration/ Perfusion*: MM pink and moist with a CRT of 1-2 sec
☐*Eyes*: No abnormalities
☐*Nose*: No abnormalities
☐*Ears*: No abnormalities; ☐Debris (mild / mod / sev) (AU / AD / AS)
☐*Oral cavity*: No abnormalities; ☐Tarter (mild / mod/ sev); ☐Gingivitis
☐*Lymph nodes*: Small, symmetrical, smooth, and soft
☐*Abdomen*: Soft, non-painful, no fluid-wave, organomegaly, or masses
☐*Mammary Chain*: No abnormalities
☐*Penis/ Vulva*: No abnormalities
☐*Skin*: No alopecia, masses, erythema, other lesions, or ectoparasites
☐*Neuro*: No paresis, ataxia, or postural deficits, normal PLR and mentation
☐*MS*: Adequate and symmetrical muscling, no overt lameness
☐*Rectal*: No abnormalities, normal colored feces on glove

Labwork:

Other Diagnostics:
Blood Pressure:

Problem List:

Plan:

Case No._____

Patient		Age	Sex	Breed		Weight
		DOB:	Mn / Mi Fs / Fi	Color:		kg

Owner		Primary Veterinarian	Admit Date/ Time
Name: Phone:		Name: Phone:	Date: Time: AM / PM

• **Presenting Complaint**:_____

• **Medical Hx**:_____

• **When/ where obtained**:   Date:_____; ☐Breeder, ☐Shelter, Other:_____

Drug/ Suppl.	Amount	Dose (mg/kg)	Route	Frequency	Date Started

• **Vaccine status – Dog**: ☐Rab ☐Parv ☐Dist ☐Aden; ☐Para ☐Lep ☐Bord ☐Influ ☐Lyme
• **Vaccine status – Cat**: ☐Rab ☐Herp ☐Cali ☐Pan ☐FeLV[kittens]; ☐FIV ☐Chlam ☐Bord
• **Heartworm / Flea & Tick / Intestinal Parasites**:
  ◦ *Last Heartworm Test*: Date:_____, ☐IDK; Test Results: ☐Pos, ☐Neg, ☐IDK
  ◦ *Monthly heartworm preventative*: ☐no ☐yes, Product:_____
  ◦ *Monthly flea & tick preventative*: ☐no ☐yes, Product:_____
  ◦ *Monthly dewormer*: ☐no ☐yes, Product:_____
• **Surgical Hx**: ☐Spay/Neuter; Date:_____; Other:_____
• **Environment**: ☐Indoor, ☐Outdoor, Time spent outdoors/ Other:_____
• **Housemates**: Dogs:_____ Cats:_____ Other:_____
• **Diet**: ☐Wet, ☐Dry; Brand/ Amt.:_____

Appetite	☐Normal, ☐↑, ☐↓
Weight	☐Normal, ☐↑, ☐↓; Past Wt.:_____ kg; Date:_____; Δ:_____
Thirst	☐Normal, ☐↑, ☐↓
Urination	☐Normal, ☐↑, ☐↓, ☐Blood, ☐Strain
Defecation	☐Normal, ☐↑, ☐↓, ☐Blood, ☐Strain, ☐Diarrhea, ☐Mucus
Discharge	☐No, ☐Yes; Onset/ Describe:
Cough/ Sneeze	☐No, ☐Yes; Onset/ Describe:
Vomit	☐No, ☐Yes; Onset/ Describe:
Respiration	☐Normal, ☐↑ Rate, ☐↑ Effort
Energy level	☐Normal, ☐Lethargic, ☐Exercise intolerance

• **Travel Hx**: ☐None, Other:_____
• **Exposure to**: ☐Standing water, ☐Wildlife, ☐Board/daycare, ☐Dog park, ☐Groomer
• **Adverse reactions to food/ meds**: ☐None, Other:_____
• Can give oral meds: ☐no ☐yes; Helpful Tricks:_____

Physical Exam:

T:　　*P:*　　*R:*　　*Wt.:*　　*BCS:*　　*Pain:*　　*CRT:*

☐*CV*: Regular rhythm, no murmur, normokinetic and synchronous pulses
☐*Resp*: Normal BV sounds/ effort, normal tracheal sounds/ palpation
☐*Attitude*: Bright, alert, and responsive
☐*Hydration/ Perfusion*: MM pink and moist with a CRT of 1-2 sec
☐*Eyes*: No abnormalities
☐*Nose*: No abnormalities
☐*Ears*: No abnormalities; ☐Debris (mild / mod / sev) (AU / AD / AS)
☐*Oral cavity*: No abnormalities; ☐Tarter (mild / mod/ sev); ☐Gingivitis
☐*Lymph nodes*: Small, symmetrical, smooth, and soft
☐*Abdomen*: Soft, non-painful, no fluid-wave, organomegaly, or masses
☐*Mammary Chain*: No abnormalities
☐*Penis/ Vulva*: No abnormalities
☐*Skin*: No alopecia, masses, erythema, other lesions, or ectoparasites
☐*Neuro*: No paresis, ataxia, or postural deficits, normal PLR and mentation
☐*MS*: Adequate and symmetrical muscling, no overt lameness
☐*Rectal*: No abnormalities, normal colored feces on glove

Labwork:

Other Diagnostics:
Blood Pressure:

Problem List:

Plan:

Case No._____

Patient	Age	Sex	Breed	Weight
	DOB:	Mn / Mi Fs / Fi Color:		kg

Owner	Primary Veterinarian	Admit Date/ Time
Name: Phone:	Name: Phone:	Date: Time: AM / PM

• **Presenting Complaint**:_____

_____

• **Medical Hx**:_____

_____

• **When/ where obtained**:   Date:_____;   □Breeder, □Shelter, Other:_____

Drug/ Suppl.	Amount	Dose (mg/kg)	Route	Frequency	Date Started

• **Vaccine status – Dog**: □Rab □Parv □Dist □Aden; □Para □Lep □Bord □Influ □Lyme
• **Vaccine status – Cat**: □Rab □Herp □Cali □Pan □FeLV[kittens]; □FIV □Chlam □Bord
• **Heartworm / Flea & Tick / Intestinal Parasites**:
  ◦ *Last Heartworm Test*: Date:_____, □IDK; Test Results: □Pos, □Neg, □IDK
  ◦ *Monthly heartworm preventative*:   □no □yes, Product:_____
  ◦ *Monthly flea & tick preventative*:   □no □yes, Product:_____
  ◦ *Monthly dewormer*:   □no □yes, Product:_____
• **Surgical Hx**:   □Spay/Neuter; Date:_____;   Other:_____
• **Environment**: □Indoor, □Outdoor, Time spent outdoors/ Other:_____
• **Housemates**: Dogs:_____ Cats:_____ Other:_____
• **Diet**: □Wet, □Dry; Brand/ Amt.:_____

Appetite	□Normal, □↑, □↓
Weight	□Normal, □↑, □↓; Past Wt.:_____kg; Date:_____; Δ:_____
Thirst	□Normal, □↑, □↓
Urination	□Normal, □↑, □↓, □Blood, □Strain
Defecation	□Normal, □↑, □↓, □Blood, □Strain, □Diarrhea, □Mucus
Discharge	□No, □Yes; Onset/ Describe:
Cough/ Sneeze	□No, □Yes; Onset/ Describe:
Vomit	□No, □Yes; Onset/ Describe:
Respiration	□Normal, □↑ Rate, □↑ Effort
Energy level	□Normal, □Lethargic, □Exercise intolerance

• **Travel Hx**: □None, Other:_____
• **Exposure to**: □Standing water, □Wildlife, □Board/daycare, □Dog park, □Groomer
• **Adverse reactions to food/ meds**: □None, Other:_____
• Can give oral meds: □no □yes; Helpful Tricks:_____

Physical Exam:

T: *P:*   *R:*   *Wt.:*   *BCS:*   *Pain:*   *CRT:*

☐*CV*: Regular rhythm, no murmur, normokinetic and synchronous pulses
☐*Resp*: Normal BV sounds/ effort, normal tracheal sounds/ palpation
☐*Attitude*: Bright, alert, and responsive
☐*Hydration/ Perfusion*: MM pink and moist with a CRT of 1-2 sec
☐*Eyes*: No abnormalities
☐*Nose*: No abnormalities
☐*Ears*: No abnormalities; ☐Debris (mild / mod / sev) (AU / AD / AS)
☐*Oral cavity*: No abnormalities; ☐Tarter (mild / mod/ sev); ☐Gingivitis
☐*Lymph nodes*: Small, symmetrical, smooth, and soft
☐*Abdomen*: Soft, non-painful, no fluid-wave, organomegaly, or masses
☐*Mammary Chain*: No abnormalities
☐*Penis/ Vulva*: No abnormalities
☐*Skin*: No alopecia, masses, erythema, other lesions, or ectoparasites
☐*Neuro*: No paresis, ataxia, or postural deficits, normal PLR and mentation
☐*MS*: Adequate and symmetrical muscling, no overt lameness
☐*Rectal*: No abnormalities, normal colored feces on glove

Labwork:

Other Diagnostics:
Blood Pressure:

Problem List:

Plan:

Patient	Age	Sex	Breed	Weight
	DOB:	Mn / Mi Fs / Fi	Color:	k

Owner	Primary Veterinarian	Admit Date/ Time
Name: Phone:	Name: Phone:	Date: Time: AM / PM

- **Presenting Complaint**:_____

- **Medical Hx**:_____

- **When/ where obtained**:   Date:_____ ; □Breeder, □Shelter, Other:_____

Drug/ Suppl.	Amount	Dose (mg/kg)	Route	Frequency	Date Started

- **Vaccine status – Dog**: □Rab □Parv □Dist □Aden; □Para □Lep □Bord □Influ □Lyme
- **Vaccine status – Cat**: □Rab □Herp □Cali □Pan □FeLV[kittens]; □FIV □Chlam □Bord
- **Heartworm / Flea & Tick / Intestinal Parasites**:
  - *Last Heartworm Test*: Date:_____, □IDK; Test Results: □Pos, □Neg, □IDK
  - *Monthly heartworm preventative*:   □no □yes,   Product:_____
  - *Monthly flea & tick preventative*:   □no □yes,   Product:_____
  - *Monthly dewormer*:   □no □yes,   Product:_____
- **Surgical Hx**:   □Spay/Neuter; Date:_____ ;   Other:_____
- **Environment**: □Indoor, □Outdoor, Time spent outdoors/ Other:_____
- **Housemates**: Dogs:_____ Cats:_____ Other:_____
- **Diet**: □Wet, □Dry; Brand/ Amt.:_____

Appetite	□Normal, □↑, □↓
Weight	□Normal, □↑, □↓; Past Wt.:_____ kg; Date:_____ ; Δ:_____
Thirst	□Normal, □↑, □↓
Urination	□Normal, □↑, □↓, □Blood, □Strain
Defecation	□Normal, □↑, □↓, □Blood, □Strain, □Diarrhea, □Mucus
Discharge	□No, □Yes; Onset/ Describe:
Cough/ Sneeze	□No, □Yes; Onset/ Describe:
Vomit	□No, □Yes; Onset/ Describe:
Respiration	□Normal, □↑ Rate, □↑ Effort
Energy level	□Normal, □Lethargic, □Exercise intolerance

- **Travel Hx**: □None, Other:_____
- **Exposure to**: □Standing water, □Wildlife, □Board/daycare, □Dog park, □Groomer
- **Adverse reactions to food/ meds**: □None, Other:_____
- Can give oral meds: □no □yes; Helpful Tricks:_____

Physical Exam:

T: *P*:   *R*:   *Wt.*:   *BCS*:   *Pain*:   *CRT*:

☐*CV*: Regular rhythm, no murmur, normokinetic and synchronous pulses
☐*Resp*: Normal BV sounds/ effort, normal tracheal sounds/ palpation
☐*Attitude*: Bright, alert, and responsive
☐*Hydration/ Perfusion*: MM pink and moist with a CRT of 1-2 sec
☐*Eyes*: No abnormalities
☐*Nose*: No abnormalities
☐*Ears*: No abnormalities; ☐Debris (mild / mod / sev) (AU / AD / AS)
☐*Oral cavity*: No abnormalities; ☐Tarter (mild / mod/ sev); ☐Gingivitis
☐*Lymph nodes*: Small, symmetrical, smooth, and soft
☐*Abdomen*: Soft, non-painful, no fluid-wave, organomegaly, or masses
☐*Mammary Chain*: No abnormalities
☐*Penis/ Vulva*: No abnormalities
☐*Skin*: No alopecia, masses, erythema, other lesions, or ectoparasites
☐*Neuro*: No paresis, ataxia, or postural deficits, normal PLR and mentation
☐*MS*: Adequate and symmetrical muscling, no overt lameness
☐*Rectal*: No abnormalities, normal colored feces on glove

Labwork:

Other Diagnostics:
Blood Pressure:

Problem List:

Plan:

Patient	Age	Sex	Breed	Weight
	DOB:	Mn / Mi Fs / Fi	Color:	kg

Owner	Primary Veterinarian	Admit Date/ Time
Name: Phone:	Name: Phone:	Date: Time: ___ AM / PM

• **Presenting Complaint**:_____
_____
_____

• **Medical Hx**:_____
_____
_____

• **When/ where obtained**: Date:_____ ; □Breeder, □Shelter, Other:_____

Drug/ Suppl.	Amount	Dose (mg/kg)	Route	Frequency	Date Started

• **Vaccine status – Dog**: □Rab □Parv □Dist □Aden; □Para □Lep □Bord □Influ □Lyme
• **Vaccine status – Cat**: □Rab □Herp □Cali □Pan □FeLV[kittens]; □FIV □Chlam □Bord
• **Heartworm / Flea & Tick / Intestinal Parasites**:
  ◦ *Last Heartworm Test*: Date:_____, □IDK; Test Results: □Pos, □Neg, □IDK
  ◦ *Monthly heartworm preventative*: □no □yes, Product:_____
  ◦ *Monthly flea & tick preventative*: □no □yes, Product:_____
  ◦ *Monthly dewormer*: □no □yes, Product:_____
• **Surgical Hx**: □Spay/Neuter; Date:_____; Other:_____
• **Environment**: □Indoor, □Outdoor, Time spent outdoors/ Other:_____
• **Housemates**: Dogs:_____ Cats:_____ Other:_____
• **Diet**: □Wet, □Dry; Brand/ Amt.:_____

Appetite	□Normal, □↑, □↓
Weight	□Normal, □↑, □↓; Past Wt.:_____ kg; Date:_____ ; Δ:_____
Thirst	□Normal, □↑, □↓
Urination	□Normal, □↑, □↓, □Blood, □Strain
Defecation	□Normal, □↑, □↓, □Blood, □Strain, □Diarrhea, □Mucus
Discharge	□No, □Yes; Onset/ Describe:
Cough/ Sneeze	□No, □Yes; Onset/ Describe:
Vomit	□No, □Yes; Onset/ Describe:
Respiration	□Normal, □↑ Rate, □↑ Effort
Energy level	□Normal, □Lethargic, □Exercise intolerance

• **Travel Hx**: □None, Other:_____
• **Exposure to**: □Standing water, □Wildlife, □Board/daycare, □Dog park, □Groomer
• **Adverse reactions to food/ meds**: □None, Other:_____
• **Can give oral meds**: □no □yes; Helpful Tricks:_____

Physical Exam:

T: *P:*   *R:*   *Wt.:*   *BCS:*   *Pain:*   *CRT:*

☐*CV*: Regular rhythm, no murmur, normokinetic and synchronous pulses
☐*Resp*: Normal BV sounds/ effort, normal tracheal sounds/ palpation
☐*Attitude*: Bright, alert, and responsive
☐*Hydration/ Perfusion*: MM pink and moist with a CRT of 1-2 sec
☐*Eyes*: No abnormalities
☐*Nose*: No abnormalities
☐*Ears*: No abnormalities; ☐Debris (mild / mod / sev) (AU / AD / AS)
☐*Oral cavity*: No abnormalities; ☐Tarter (mild / mod/ sev); ☐Gingivitis
☐*Lymph nodes*: Small, symmetrical, smooth, and soft
☐*Abdomen*: Soft, non-painful, no fluid-wave, organomegaly, or masses
☐*Mammary Chain*: No abnormalities
☐*Penis/ Vulva*: No abnormalities
☐*Skin*: No alopecia, masses, erythema, other lesions, or ectoparasites
☐*Neuro*: No paresis, ataxia, or postural deficits, normal PLR and mentation
☐*MS*: Adequate and symmetrical muscling, no overt lameness
☐*Rectal*: No abnormalities, normal colored feces on glove

Labwork:

Other Diagnostics:
Blood Pressure:

Problem List:

Plan:

Patient	Age	Sex	Breed	Weight
	DOB:	Mn / Mi Fs / Fi	Color:	kg

Owner	Primary Veterinarian	Admit Date/ Time
Name: Phone:	Name: Phone:	Date: Time: AM / PM

• **Presenting Complaint**:_____
_____
_____

• **Medical Hx**:_____
_____
_____

• **When/ where obtained**: Date:_____; □Breeder, □Shelter, Other:_____

Drug/ Suppl.	Amount	Dose (mg/kg)	Route	Frequency	Date Started

• **Vaccine status – Dog**: □Rab □Parv □Dist □Aden; □Para □Lep □Bord □Influ □Lyme
• **Vaccine status – Cat**: □Rab □Herp □Cali □Pan □FeLV[kittens]; □FIV □Chlam □Bord
• **Heartworm / Flea & Tick / Intestinal Parasites**:
  ◦ *Last Heartworm Test*: Date:_____, □IDK; Test Results: □Pos, □Neg, □IDK
  ◦ *Monthly heartworm preventative*: □no □yes, Product:_____
  ◦ *Monthly flea & tick preventative*: □no □yes, Product:_____
  ◦ *Monthly dewormer*: □no □yes, Product:_____
• **Surgical Hx**: □Spay/Neuter; Date:_____; Other:_____
• **Environment**: □Indoor, □Outdoor, Time spent outdoors/ Other:_____
• **Housemates**: Dogs:_____ Cats:_____ Other:_____
• **Diet**: □Wet, □Dry; Brand/ Amt.:_____

Appetite	□Normal, □↑, □↓
Weight	□Normal, □↑, □↓; Past Wt.:_____ kg; Date:_____; Δ:_____
Thirst	□Normal, □↑, □↓
Urination	□Normal, □↑, □↓, □Blood, □Strain
Defecation	□Normal, □↑, □↓, □Blood, □Strain, □Diarrhea, □Mucus
Discharge	□No, □Yes; Onset/ Describe:
Cough/ Sneeze	□No, □Yes; Onset/ Describe:
Vomit	□No, □Yes; Onset/ Describe:
Respiration	□Normal, □↑ Rate, □↑ Effort
Energy level	□Normal, □Lethargic, □Exercise intolerance

• **Travel Hx**: □None, Other:_____
• **Exposure to**: □Standing water, □Wildlife, □Board/daycare, □Dog park, □Groomer
• **Adverse reactions to food/ meds**: □None, Other:_____
• Can give oral meds: □no □yes; Helpful Tricks:_____

Physical Exam:

T: *P:*   *R:*   *Wt.:*   *BCS:*   *Pain:*   *CRT:*

☐*CV*: Regular rhythm, no murmur, normokinetic and synchronous pulses
☐*Resp*: Normal BV sounds/ effort, normal tracheal sounds/ palpation
☐*Attitude*: Bright, alert, and responsive
☐*Hydration/ Perfusion*: MM pink and moist with a CRT of 1-2 sec
☐*Eyes*: No abnormalities
☐*Nose*: No abnormalities
☐*Ears*: No abnormalities; ☐Debris (mild / mod / sev) (AU / AD / AS)
☐*Oral cavity*: No abnormalities; ☐Tarter (mild / mod/ sev); ☐Gingivitis
☐*Lymph nodes*: Small, symmetrical, smooth, and soft
☐*Abdomen*: Soft, non-painful, no fluid-wave, organomegaly, or masses
☐*Mammary Chain*: No abnormalities
☐*Penis/ Vulva*: No abnormalities
☐*Skin*: No alopecia, masses, erythema, other lesions, or ectoparasites
☐*Neuro*: No paresis, ataxia, or postural deficits, normal PLR and mentation
☐*MS*: Adequate and symmetrical muscling, no overt lameness
☐*Rectal*: No abnormalities, normal colored feces on glove

Labwork:

Other Diagnostics:
Blood Pressure:

Problem List:

Plan:

Case No._____

Patient	Age	Sex	Breed	Weigh
	DOB:	Mn / Mi Fs / Fi	Color:	k

Owner		Primary Veterinarian	Admit Date/ Time
Name: Phone:		Name: Phone:	Date: Time: AM / PM

- **Presenting Complaint**:_____
  _____
  _____

- **Medical Hx**:_____
  _____
  _____

- **When/ where obtained**:   Date:_____; □Breeder, □Shelter, Other:_____

Drug/ Suppl.	Amount	Dose (mg/kg)	Route	Frequency	Date Started

- **Vaccine status – Dog**: □Rab □Parv □Dist □Aden; □Para □Lep □Bord □Influ □Lyme
- **Vaccine status – Cat**: □Rab □Herp □Cali □Pan □FeLV[kittens]; □FIV □Chlam □Bord
- **Heartworm / Flea & Tick / Intestinal Parasites**:
  - *Last Heartworm Test*: Date:_____, □IDK; Test Results: □Pos, □Neg, □IDK
  - *Monthly heartworm preventative*: □no □yes, Product:_____
  - *Monthly flea & tick preventative*: □no □yes, Product:_____
  - *Monthly dewormer*:   □no □yes, Product:_____
- **Surgical Hx**: □Spay/Neuter; Date:_____; Other:_____
- **Environment**: □Indoor, □Outdoor, Time spent outdoors/ Other:_____
- **Housemates**: Dogs:_____ Cats:_____ Other:_____
- **Diet**: □Wet, □Dry; Brand/ Amt.:_____

Appetite	□Normal, □↑, □↓
Weight	□Normal, □↑, □↓; Past Wt.:_____ kg; Date:_____; Δ:_____
Thirst	□Normal, □↑, □↓
Urination	□Normal, □↑, □↓, □Blood, □Strain
Defecation	□Normal, □↑, □↓, □Blood, □Strain, □Diarrhea, □Mucus
Discharge	□No, □Yes; Onset/ Describe:
Cough/ Sneeze	□No, □Yes; Onset/ Describe:
Vomit	□No, □Yes; Onset/ Describe:
Respiration	□Normal, □↑ Rate, □↑ Effort
Energy level	□Normal, □Lethargic, □Exercise intolerance

- **Travel Hx**: □None, Other:_____
- **Exposure to**: □Standing water, □Wildlife, □Board/daycare, □Dog park, □Groomer
- **Adverse reactions to food/ meds**: □None, Other:_____
- Can give oral meds: □no □yes; Helpful Tricks:_____

Physical Exam:

T: *P*:   *R*:   *Wt.*:   *BCS*:   *Pain*:   *CRT*:

☐*CV*: Regular rhythm, no murmur, normokinetic and synchronous pulses
☐*Resp*: Normal BV sounds/ effort, normal tracheal sounds/ palpation
☐*Attitude*: Bright, alert, and responsive
☐*Hydration/ Perfusion*: MM pink and moist with a CRT of 1-2 sec
☐*Eyes*: No abnormalities
☐*Nose*: No abnormalities
☐*Ears*: No abnormalities; ☐Debris (mild / mod / sev) (AU / AD / AS)
☐*Oral cavity*: No abnormalities; ☐Tarter (mild / mod/ sev); ☐Gingivitis
☐*Lymph nodes*: Small, symmetrical, smooth, and soft
☐*Abdomen*: Soft, non-painful, no fluid-wave, organomegaly, or masses
☐*Mammary Chain*: No abnormalities
☐*Penis/ Vulva*: No abnormalities
☐*Skin*: No alopecia, masses, erythema, other lesions, or ectoparasites
☐*Neuro*: No paresis, ataxia, or postural deficits, normal PLR and mentation
☐*MS*: Adequate and symmetrical muscling, no overt lameness
☐*Rectal*: No abnormalities, normal colored feces on glove

Labwork:

Other Diagnostics:
Blood Pressure:

Problem List:

Plan:

Case No._____

Patient	Age	Sex	Breed	Weight
	DOB:	Mn / Mi Fs / Fi	Color:	kg

Owner		Primary Veterinarian	Admit Date/ Time
Name: Phone:		Name: Phone:	Date: Time: AM / PM

• **Presenting Complaint**:_____
_____
_____

• **Medical Hx**:_____
_____
_____

• **When/ where obtained**:   Date:_____; □Breeder, □Shelter, Other:_____

Drug/ Suppl.	Amount	Dose (mg/kg)	Route	Frequency	Date Started

• **Vaccine status – Dog**: □Rab □Parv □Dist □Aden; □Para □Lep □Bord □Influ □Lyme
• **Vaccine status – Cat**: □Rab □Herp □Cali □Pan □FeLV[kittens]; □FIV □Chlam □Bord
• **Heartworm / Flea & Tick / Intestinal Parasites**:
  ◦ *Last Heartworm Test*: Date:_____, □IDK; Test Results: □Pos, □Neg, □IDK
  ◦ *Monthly heartworm preventative*: □no □yes, Product:_____
  ◦ *Monthly flea & tick preventative*: □no □yes, Product:_____
  ◦ *Monthly dewormer*:   □no □yes, Product:_____
• **Surgical Hx**: □Spay/Neuter; Date:_____; Other:_____
• **Environment**: □Indoor, □Outdoor, Time spent outdoors/ Other:_____
• **Housemates**: Dogs:_____ Cats:_____ Other:_____
• **Diet**: □Wet, □Dry; Brand/ Amt.:_____

Appetite	□Normal, □↑, □↓
Weight	□Normal, □↑, □↓; Past Wt.:_____ kg; Date:_____; Δ:_____
Thirst	□Normal, □↑, □↓
Urination	□Normal, □↑, □↓, □Blood, □Strain
Defecation	□Normal, □↑, □↓, □Blood, □Strain, □Diarrhea, □Mucus
Discharge	□No, □Yes; Onset/ Describe:
Cough/ Sneeze	□No, □Yes; Onset/ Describe:
Vomit	□No, □Yes; Onset/ Describe:
Respiration	□Normal, □↑ Rate, □↑ Effort
Energy level	□Normal, □Lethargic, □Exercise intolerance

• **Travel Hx**: □None, Other:_____
• **Exposure to**: □Standing water, □Wildlife, □Board/daycare, □Dog park, □Groomer
• **Adverse reactions to food/ meds**: □None, Other:_____
• Can give oral meds: □no □yes; Helpful Tricks:_____

Physical Exam:

T: P: R: Wt.:   BCS: Pain: CRT:

☐*CV*: Regular rhythm, no murmur, normokinetic and synchronous pulses
☐*Resp*: Normal BV sounds/ effort, normal tracheal sounds/ palpation
☐*Attitude*: Bright, alert, and responsive
☐*Hydration/ Perfusion*: MM pink and moist with a CRT of 1-2 sec
☐*Eyes*: No abnormalities
☐*Nose*: No abnormalities
☐*Ears*: No abnormalities; ☐Debris (mild / mod / sev) (AU / AD / AS)
☐*Oral cavity*: No abnormalities; ☐Tarter (mild / mod/ sev); ☐Gingivitis
☐*Lymph nodes*: Small, symmetrical, smooth, and soft
☐*Abdomen*: Soft, non-painful, no fluid-wave, organomegaly, or masses
☐*Mammary Chain*: No abnormalities
☐*Penis/ Vulva*: No abnormalities
☐*Skin*: No alopecia, masses, erythema, other lesions, or ectoparasites
☐*Neuro*: No paresis, ataxia, or postural deficits, normal PLR and mentation
☐*MS*: Adequate and symmetrical muscling, no overt lameness
☐*Rectal*: No abnormalities, normal colored feces on glove

Labwork:

Other Diagnostics:
Blood Pressure:

Problem List:

Plan:

Case No._____

Patient	Age	Sex	Breed	Weight
	DOB:	Mn / Mi Fs / Fi	Color:	kg

Owner	Primary Veterinarian	Admit Date/ Time
Name: Phone:	Name: Phone:	Date: Time: AM / PM

• **Presenting Complaint**:_____

_____

_____

• **Medical Hx**:_____

_____

_____

• **When/ where obtained**:   Date:_____; ☐Breeder, ☐Shelter, Other:_____

Drug/ Suppl.	Amount	Dose (mg/kg)	Route	Frequency	Date Started

• **Vaccine status – Dog**: ☐Rab ☐Parv ☐Dist ☐Aden; ☐Para ☐Lep ☐Bord ☐Influ ☐Lyme
• **Vaccine status – Cat**: ☐Rab ☐Herp ☐Cali ☐Pan ☐FeLV[kittens]; ☐FIV ☐Chlam ☐Bord
• **Heartworm / Flea & Tick / Intestinal Parasites**:
   ◦ *Last Heartworm Test*: Date:_____, ☐IDK; Test Results: ☐Pos, ☐Neg, ☐IDK
   ◦ *Monthly heartworm preventative*:   ☐no ☐yes, Product:_____
   ◦ *Monthly flea & tick preventative*: ☐no ☐yes, Product:_____
   ◦ *Monthly dewormer*:   ☐no ☐yes, Product:_____
• **Surgical Hx**:   ☐Spay/Neuter; Date:_____; Other:_____
• **Environment**: ☐Indoor, ☐Outdoor, Time spent outdoors/ Other:_____
• **Housemates**: Dogs:_____ Cats:_____ Other:_____
• **Diet**: ☐Wet, ☐Dry; Brand/ Amt.:_____

Appetite	☐Normal, ☐↑, ☐↓
Weight	☐Normal, ☐↑, ☐↓; Past Wt.:_____ kg; Date:_____; Δ:_____
Thirst	☐Normal, ☐↑, ☐↓
Urination	☐Normal, ☐↑, ☐↓, ☐Blood, ☐Strain
Defecation	☐Normal, ☐↑, ☐↓, ☐Blood, ☐Strain, ☐Diarrhea, ☐Mucus
Discharge	☐No, ☐Yes; Onset/ Describe:
Cough/ Sneeze	☐No, ☐Yes; Onset/ Describe:
Vomit	☐No, ☐Yes; Onset/ Describe:
Respiration	☐Normal, ☐↑ Rate, ☐↑ Effort
Energy level	☐Normal, ☐Lethargic, ☐Exercise intolerance

• **Travel Hx**: ☐None, Other:_____
• **Exposure to**: ☐Standing water, ☐Wildlife, ☐Board/daycare, ☐Dog park, ☐Groomer
• **Adverse reactions to food/ meds**: ☐None, Other:_____
• Can give oral meds: ☐no ☐yes; Helpful Tricks:_____

Physical Exam:

*:   P: R: Wt.:   BCS: Pain: CRT:

]*CV*: Regular rhythm, no murmur, normokinetic and synchronous pulses
]*Resp*: Normal BV sounds/ effort, normal tracheal sounds/ palpation
]*Attitude*: Bright, alert, and responsive
]*Hydration/ Perfusion*: MM pink and moist with a CRT of 1-2 sec
]*Eyes*: No abnormalities
]*Nose*: No abnormalities
]*Ears*: No abnormalities; ☐Debris (mild / mod / sev) (AU / AD / AS)
]*Oral cavity*: No abnormalities; ☐Tarter (mild / mod/ sev); ☐Gingivitis
]*Lymph nodes*: Small, symmetrical, smooth, and soft
]*Abdomen*: Soft, non-painful, no fluid-wave, organomegaly, or masses
]*Mammary Chain*: No abnormalities
]*Penis/ Vulva*: No abnormalities
]*Skin*: No alopecia, masses, erythema, other lesions, or ectoparasites
]*Neuro*: No paresis, ataxia, or postural deficits, normal PLR and mentation
]*MS*: Adequate and symmetrical muscling, no overt lameness
]*Rectal*: No abnormalities, normal colored feces on glove

abwork:

Other Diagnostics:
Blood Pressure:

roblem List:

lan:

Case No._____

Patient	Age	Sex	Breed	Weight
	DOB:	Mn / Mi Fs / Fi	Color:	k

Owner		Primary Veterinarian	Admit Date/ Time
Name: Phone:		Name: Phone:	Date: Time: AM / PM

• **Presenting Complaint**: _____
_____
_____

• **Medical Hx**: _____
_____
_____

• **When/ where obtained**:   Date:_____ ; ☐Breeder, ☐Shelter, Other:_____

Drug/ Suppl.	Amount	Dose (mg/kg)	Route	Frequency	Date Started

• **Vaccine status – Dog**: ☐Rab ☐Parv ☐Dist ☐Aden; ☐Para ☐Lep ☐Bord ☐Influ ☐Lyme
• **Vaccine status – Cat**: ☐Rab ☐Herp ☐Cali ☐Pan ☐FeLV[kittens]; ☐FIV ☐Chlam ☐Bord
• **Heartworm / Flea & Tick / Intestinal Parasites**:
  ○ *Last Heartworm Test*: Date:_____ , ☐IDK; Test Results: ☐Pos, ☐Neg, ☐IDK
  ○ *Monthly heartworm preventative*: ☐no ☐yes, Product:_____
  ○ *Monthly flea & tick preventative*: ☐no ☐yes, Product:_____
  ○ *Monthly dewormer*: ☐no ☐yes, Product:_____
• **Surgical Hx**: ☐Spay/Neuter; Date:_____ ; Other:_____
• **Environment**: ☐Indoor, ☐Outdoor, Time spent outdoors/ Other:_____
• **Housemates**: Dogs:_____ Cats:_____ Other:_____
• **Diet**: ☐Wet, ☐Dry; Brand/ Amt.:_____

Appetite	☐Normal, ☐↑, ☐↓
Weight	☐Normal, ☐↑, ☐↓; Past Wt.:_____ kg; Date:_____ ; Δ:_____
Thirst	☐Normal, ☐↑, ☐↓
Urination	☐Normal, ☐↑, ☐↓, ☐Blood, ☐Strain
Defecation	☐Normal, ☐↑, ☐↓, ☐Blood, ☐Strain, ☐Diarrhea, ☐Mucus
Discharge	☐No, ☐Yes; Onset/ Describe:
Cough/ Sneeze	☐No, ☐Yes; Onset/ Describe:
Vomit	☐No, ☐Yes; Onset/ Describe:
Respiration	☐Normal, ☐↑ Rate, ☐↑ Effort
Energy level	☐Normal, ☐Lethargic, ☐Exercise intolerance

• **Travel Hx**: ☐None, Other:_____
• **Exposure to**: ☐Standing water, ☐Wildlife, ☐Board/daycare, ☐Dog park, ☐Groomer
• **Adverse reactions to food/ meds**: ☐None, Other:_____
• Can give oral meds: ☐no ☐yes; Helpful Tricks:_____

Physical Exam:

T: P: R: Wt.:   BCS: Pain: CRT:

☐*CV*: Regular rhythm, no murmur, normokinetic and synchronous pulses
☐*Resp*: Normal BV sounds/ effort, normal tracheal sounds/ palpation
☐*Attitude*: Bright, alert, and responsive
☐*Hydration/ Perfusion*: MM pink and moist with a CRT of 1-2 sec
☐*Eyes*: No abnormalities
☐*Nose*: No abnormalities
☐*Ears*: No abnormalities; ☐Debris (mild / mod / sev) (AU / AD / AS)
☐*Oral cavity*: No abnormalities; ☐Tarter (mild / mod/ sev); ☐Gingivitis
☐*Lymph nodes*: Small, symmetrical, smooth, and soft
☐*Abdomen*: Soft, non-painful, no fluid-wave, organomegaly, or masses
☐*Mammary Chain*: No abnormalities
☐*Penis/ Vulva*: No abnormalities
☐*Skin*: No alopecia, masses, erythema, other lesions, or ectoparasites
☐*Neuro*: No paresis, ataxia, or postural deficits, normal PLR and mentation
☐*MS*: Adequate and symmetrical muscling, no overt lameness
☐*Rectal*: No abnormalities, normal colored feces on glove

Labwork:	**Other Diagnostics:**
	Blood Pressure:

Problem List:

Plan:

Case No._____

Patient	Age	Sex	Breed	Weight
	DOB:	Mn / Mi Fs / Fi	Color:	kg

Owner	Primary Veterinarian	Admit Date/ Time
Name: Phone:	Name: Phone:	Date: Time:　　AM / PM

• **Presenting Complaint**:_____

_____

• **Medical Hx**:_____

_____

• **When/ where obtained**:　Date:_____; □Breeder, □Shelter, Other:_____

Drug/ Suppl.	Amount	Dose (mg/kg)	Route	Frequency	Date Started

• **Vaccine status – Dog**: □Rab □Parv □Dist □Aden; □Para □Lep □Bord □Influ □Lyme
• **Vaccine status – Cat**: □Rab □Herp □Cali □Pan □FeLV[kittens]; □FIV □Chlam □Bord
• **Heartworm / Flea & Tick / Intestinal Parasites**:
　　○ *Last Heartworm Test*: Date:_____, □IDK;　Test Results: □Pos, □Neg, □IDK
　　○ *Monthly heartworm preventative*:　□no □yes,　Product:_____
　　○ *Monthly flea & tick preventative*:　□no □yes,　Product:_____
　　○ *Monthly dewormer*:　　　　　　　□no □yes,　Product:_____
• **Surgical Hx**:　□Spay/Neuter; Date:_____;　Other:_____
• **Environment**:　□Indoor, □Outdoor,　Time spent outdoors/ Other:_____
• **Housemates**:　Dogs:_____　Cats:_____　Other:_____
• **Diet**: □Wet, □Dry; Brand/ Amt.:_____

Appetite	□Normal, □↑, □↓
Weight	□Normal, □↑, □↓; Past Wt.:_____ kg; Date:_____; Δ:_____
Thirst	□Normal, □↑, □↓
Urination	□Normal, □↑, □↓, □Blood, □Strain
Defecation	□Normal, □↑, □↓, □Blood, □Strain, □Diarrhea, □Mucus
Discharge	□No, □Yes; Onset/ Describe:
Cough/ Sneeze	□No, □Yes; Onset/ Describe:
Vomit	□No, □Yes; Onset/ Describe:
Respiration	□Normal, □↑ Rate, □↑ Effort
Energy level	□Normal, □Lethargic, □Exercise intolerance

• **Travel Hx**: □None, Other:_____
• **Exposure to**: □Standing water, □Wildlife, □Board/daycare, □Dog park, □Groomer
• **Adverse reactions to food/ meds**: □None, Other:_____
• Can give oral meds: □no □yes; Helpful Tricks:_____

Physical Exam:

T: P: R: Wt.:   BCS: Pain: CRT:

☐*CV*: Regular rhythm, no murmur, normokinetic and synchronous pulses
☐*Resp*: Normal BV sounds/ effort, normal tracheal sounds/ palpation
☐*Attitude*: Bright, alert, and responsive
☐*Hydration/ Perfusion*: MM pink and moist with a CRT of 1-2 sec
☐*Eyes*: No abnormalities
☐*Nose*: No abnormalities
☐*Ears*: No abnormalities; ☐Debris (mild / mod / sev) (AU / AD / AS)
☐*Oral cavity*: No abnormalities; ☐Tarter (mild / mod/ sev); ☐Gingivitis
☐*Lymph nodes*: Small, symmetrical, smooth, and soft
☐*Abdomen*: Soft, non-painful, no fluid-wave, organomegaly, or masses
☐*Mammary Chain*: No abnormalities
☐*Penis/ Vulva*: No abnormalities
☐*Skin*: No alopecia, masses, erythema, other lesions, or ectoparasites
☐*Neuro*: No paresis, ataxia, or postural deficits, normal PLR and mentation
☐*MS*: Adequate and symmetrical muscling, no overt lameness
☐*Rectal*: No abnormalities, normal colored feces on glove

Labwork:

Other Diagnostics:
Blood Pressure:

Problem List:

Plan:

Case No._____

Patient	Age	Sex	Breed	Weight
	DOB:	Mn / Mi Fs / Fi	Color:	kg

Owner	Primary Veterinarian	Admit Date/ Time
Name: Phone:	Name: Phone:	Date: Time: AM / PM

• **Presenting Complaint**:_____
_____
_____

• **Medical Hx**:_____
_____
_____

• **When/ where obtained**: Date:_____; □Breeder, □Shelter, Other:_____

Drug/ Suppl.	Amount	Dose (mg/kg)	Route	Frequency	Date Started

• **Vaccine status – Dog**: □Rab □Parv □Dist □Aden; □Para □Lep □Bord □Influ □Lyme
• **Vaccine status – Cat**: □Rab □Herp □Cali □Pan □FeLV[kittens]; □FIV □Chlam □Bord
• **Heartworm / Flea & Tick / Intestinal Parasites**:
  ◦ *Last Heartworm Test*: Date:_____, □IDK; Test Results: □Pos, □Neg, □IDK
  ◦ *Monthly heartworm preventative*: □no □yes, Product:_____
  ◦ *Monthly flea & tick preventative*: □no □yes, Product:_____
  ◦ *Monthly dewormer*: □no □yes, Product:_____
• **Surgical Hx**: □Spay/Neuter; Date:_____; Other:_____
• **Environment**: □Indoor, □Outdoor, Time spent outdoors/ Other:_____
• **Housemates**: Dogs:_____ Cats:_____ Other:_____
• **Diet**: □Wet, □Dry; Brand/ Amt.:_____

Appetite	□Normal, □↑, □↓
Weight	□Normal, □↑, □↓; Past Wt.:_____ kg; Date:_____; Δ:_____
Thirst	□Normal, □↑, □↓
Urination	□Normal, □↑, □↓, □Blood, □Strain
Defecation	□Normal, □↑, □↓, □Blood, □Strain, □Diarrhea, □Mucus
Discharge	□No, □Yes; Onset/ Describe:
Cough/ Sneeze	□No, □Yes; Onset/ Describe:
Vomit	□No, □Yes; Onset/ Describe:
Respiration	□Normal, □↑ Rate, □↑ Effort
Energy level	□Normal, □Lethargic, □Exercise intolerance

• **Travel Hx**: □None, Other:_____
• **Exposure to**: □Standing water, □Wildlife, □Board/daycare, □Dog park, □Groomer
• **Adverse reactions to food/ meds**: □None, Other:_____
• Can give oral meds: □no □yes; Helpful Tricks:_____

Physical Exam:
T: *P:*   *R:*   *Wt.:*   *BCS:*   *Pain:*   *CRT:*

☐*CV*: Regular rhythm, no murmur, normokinetic and synchronous pulses
☐*Resp*: Normal BV sounds/ effort, normal tracheal sounds/ palpation
☐*Attitude*: Bright, alert, and responsive
☐*Hydration/ Perfusion*: MM pink and moist with a CRT of 1-2 sec
☐*Eyes*: No abnormalities
☐*Nose*: No abnormalities
☐*Ears*: No abnormalities; ☐Debris (mild / mod / sev) (AU / AD / AS)
☐*Oral cavity*: No abnormalities; ☐Tarter (mild / mod/ sev); ☐Gingivitis
☐*Lymph nodes*: Small, symmetrical, smooth, and soft
☐*Abdomen*: Soft, non-painful, no fluid-wave, organomegaly, or masses
☐*Mammary Chain*: No abnormalities
☐*Penis/ Vulva*: No abnormalities
☐*Skin*: No alopecia, masses, erythema, other lesions, or ectoparasites
☐*Neuro*: No paresis, ataxia, or postural deficits, normal PLR and mentation
☐*MS*: Adequate and symmetrical muscling, no overt lameness
☐*Rectal*: No abnormalities, normal colored feces on glove

Labwork:

Other Diagnostics:
Blood Pressure:

Problem List:

Plan:

Case No._____

Patient	Age	Sex	Breed	Weight
	DOB:	Mn / Mi Fs / Fi Color:		kg

Owner	Primary Veterinarian	Admit Date/ Time
Name: Phone:	Name: Phone:	Date: Time: AM / PM

• **Presenting Complaint**:_____

_____

• **Medical Hx**:_____

_____

• **When/ where obtained**: Date:_____; ☐Breeder, ☐Shelter, Other:_____

Drug/ Suppl.	Amount	Dose (mg/kg)	Route	Frequency	Date Started

• **Vaccine status – Dog**: ☐Rab ☐Parv ☐Dist ☐Aden; ☐Para ☐Lep ☐Bord ☐Influ ☐Lyme
• **Vaccine status – Cat**: ☐Rab ☐Herp ☐Cali ☐Pan ☐FeLV[kittens]; ☐FIV ☐Chlam ☐Bord
• **Heartworm / Flea & Tick / Intestinal Parasites**:
  ◦ *Last Heartworm Test*: Date:_____, ☐IDK; Test Results: ☐Pos, ☐Neg, ☐IDK
  ◦ *Monthly heartworm preventative*: ☐no ☐yes, Product:_____
  ◦ *Monthly flea & tick preventative*: ☐no ☐yes, Product:_____
  ◦ *Monthly dewormer*: ☐no ☐yes, Product:_____
• **Surgical Hx**: ☐Spay/Neuter; Date:_____; Other:_____
• **Environment**: ☐Indoor, ☐Outdoor, Time spent outdoors/ Other:_____
• **Housemates**: Dogs:_____ Cats:_____ Other:_____
• **Diet**: ☐Wet, ☐Dry; Brand/ Amt.:_____

Appetite	☐Normal, ☐↑, ☐↓
Weight	☐Normal, ☐↑, ☐↓; Past Wt.:_____ kg; Date:_____; Δ:_____
Thirst	☐Normal, ☐↑, ☐↓
Urination	☐Normal, ☐↑, ☐↓, ☐Blood, ☐Strain
Defecation	☐Normal, ☐↑, ☐↓, ☐Blood, ☐Strain, ☐Diarrhea, ☐Mucus
Discharge	☐No, ☐Yes; Onset/ Describe:
Cough/ Sneeze	☐No, ☐Yes; Onset/ Describe:
Vomit	☐No, ☐Yes; Onset/ Describe:
Respiration	☐Normal, ☐↑ Rate, ☐↑ Effort
Energy level	☐Normal, ☐Lethargic, ☐Exercise intolerance

• **Travel Hx**: ☐None, Other:_____
• **Exposure to**: ☐Standing water, ☐Wildlife, ☐Board/daycare, ☐Dog park, ☐Groomer
• **Adverse reactions to food/ meds**: ☐None, Other:_____
• **Can give oral meds**: ☐no ☐yes; Helpful Tricks:_____

Physical Exam:

T: *P:*   *R:*   *Wt.:*   *BCS:*   *Pain:*   *CRT:*

☐*CV*: Regular rhythm, no murmur, normokinetic and synchronous pulses
☐*Resp*: Normal BV sounds/ effort, normal tracheal sounds/ palpation
☐*Attitude*: Bright, alert, and responsive
☐*Hydration/ Perfusion*: MM pink and moist with a CRT of 1-2 sec
☐*Eyes*: No abnormalities
☐*Nose*: No abnormalities
☐*Ears*: No abnormalities; ☐Debris (mild / mod / sev) (AU / AD / AS)
☐*Oral cavity*: No abnormalities; ☐Tarter (mild / mod/ sev); ☐Gingivitis
☐*Lymph nodes*: Small, symmetrical, smooth, and soft
☐*Abdomen*: Soft, non-painful, no fluid-wave, organomegaly, or masses
☐*Mammary Chain*: No abnormalities
☐*Penis/ Vulva*: No abnormalities
☐*Skin*: No alopecia, masses, erythema, other lesions, or ectoparasites
☐*Neuro*: No paresis, ataxia, or postural deficits, normal PLR and mentation
☐*MS*: Adequate and symmetrical muscling, no overt lameness
☐*Rectal*: No abnormalities, normal colored feces on glove

Labwork:

Other Diagnostics:
Blood Pressure:

Problem List:

Plan:

Patient	Age	Sex	Breed	Weight
	DOB:	Mn / Mi Fs / Fi	Color:	kg

Owner		Primary Veterinarian	Admit Date/ Time
Name: Phone:		Name: Phone:	Date: Time: AM / PM

• **Presenting Complaint**:_____

_____

_____

• **Medical Hx**:_____

_____

_____

• **When/ where obtained**: Date:_____; ☐Breeder, ☐Shelter, Other:_____

Drug/ Suppl.	Amount	Dose (mg/kg)	Route	Frequency	Date Started

• **Vaccine status – Dog**: ☐Rab ☐Parv ☐Dist ☐Aden; ☐Para ☐Lep ☐Bord ☐Influ ☐Lyme
• **Vaccine status – Cat**: ☐Rab ☐Herp ☐Cali ☐Pan ☐FeLV[kittens]; ☐FIV ☐Chlam ☐Bord
• **Heartworm / Flea & Tick / Intestinal Parasites**:
   ○ *Last Heartworm Test*: Date:_____, ☐IDK; Test Results: ☐Pos, ☐Neg, ☐IDK
   ○ *Monthly heartworm preventative*: ☐no ☐yes, Product:_____
   ○ *Monthly flea & tick preventative*: ☐no ☐yes, Product:_____
   ○ *Monthly dewormer*:   ☐no ☐yes, Product:_____
• **Surgical Hx**: ☐Spay/Neuter; Date:_____; Other:_____
• **Environment**: ☐Indoor, ☐Outdoor, Time spent outdoors/ Other:_____
• **Housemates**: Dogs:_____ Cats:_____ Other:_____
• **Diet**: ☐Wet, ☐Dry; Brand/ Amt.:_____

Appetite	☐Normal, ☐↑, ☐↓
Weight	☐Normal, ☐↑, ☐↓; Past Wt.:_____ kg; Date:_____; Δ:_____
Thirst	☐Normal, ☐↑, ☐↓
Urination	☐Normal, ☐↑, ☐↓, ☐Blood, ☐Strain
Defecation	☐Normal, ☐↑, ☐↓, ☐Blood, ☐Strain, ☐Diarrhea, ☐Mucus
Discharge	☐No, ☐Yes; Onset/ Describe:
Cough/ Sneeze	☐No, ☐Yes; Onset/ Describe:
Vomit	☐No, ☐Yes; Onset/ Describe:
Respiration	☐Normal, ☐↑ Rate, ☐↑ Effort
Energy level	☐Normal, ☐Lethargic, ☐Exercise intolerance

• **Travel Hx**: ☐None, Other:_____
• **Exposure to**: ☐Standing water, ☐Wildlife, ☐Board/daycare, ☐Dog park, ☐Groomer
• **Adverse reactions to food/ meds**: ☐None, Other:_____
• **Can give oral meds**: ☐no ☐yes; Helpful Tricks:_____

Physical Exam:

T: P: R: Wt.:   BCS: Pain: CRT:

☐_CV_: Regular rhythm, no murmur, normokinetic and synchronous pulses
☐_Resp_: Normal BV sounds/ effort, normal tracheal sounds/ palpation
☐_Attitude_: Bright, alert, and responsive
☐_Hydration/ Perfusion_: MM pink and moist with a CRT of 1-2 sec
☐_Eyes_: No abnormalities
☐_Nose_: No abnormalities
☐_Ears_: No abnormalities; ☐Debris (mild / mod / sev) (AU / AD / AS)
☐_Oral cavity_: No abnormalities; ☐Tarter (mild / mod/ sev); ☐Gingivitis
☐_Lymph nodes_: Small, symmetrical, smooth, and soft
☐_Abdomen_: Soft, non-painful, no fluid-wave, organomegaly, or masses
☐_Mammary Chain_: No abnormalities
☐_Penis/ Vulva_: No abnormalities
☐_Skin_: No alopecia, masses, erythema, other lesions, or ectoparasites
☐_Neuro_: No paresis, ataxia, or postural deficits, normal PLR and mentation
☐_MS_: Adequate and symmetrical muscling, no overt lameness
☐_Rectal_: No abnormalities, normal colored feces on glove

Labwork:

Other Diagnostics:
Blood Pressure:

Problem List:

Plan:

Case No._____

Patient	Age	Sex	Breed	Weight
	DOB:	Mn / Mi Fs / Fi	Color:	kg

Owner	Primary Veterinarian	Admit Date/ Time
Name: Phone:	Name: Phone:	Date: Time: AM / PM

• **Presenting Complaint**:_____
_____
_____

• **Medical Hx**:_____
_____
_____

• **When/ where obtained**:   Date:_____; ☐Breeder, ☐Shelter, Other:_____

Drug/ Suppl.	Amount	Dose (mg/kg)	Route	Frequency	Date Started

• **Vaccine status – Dog**: ☐Rab ☐Parv ☐Dist ☐Aden; ☐Para ☐Lep ☐Bord ☐Influ ☐Lyme
• **Vaccine status – Cat**: ☐Rab ☐Herp ☐Cali ☐Pan ☐FeLV[kittens]; ☐FIV ☐Chlam ☐Bord
• **Heartworm / Flea & Tick / Intestinal Parasites**:
  ◦ *Last Heartworm Test*: Date:_____, ☐IDK; Test Results: ☐Pos, ☐Neg, ☐IDK
  ◦ *Monthly heartworm preventative*:   ☐no ☐yes,   Product:_____
  ◦ *Monthly flea & tick preventative*:   ☐no ☐yes,   Product:_____
  ◦ *Monthly dewormer*:   ☐no ☐yes,   Product:_____
• **Surgical Hx**:   ☐Spay/Neuter; Date:_____;   Other:_____
• **Environment**: ☐Indoor, ☐Outdoor, Time spent outdoors/ Other:_____
• **Housemates**: Dogs:_____ Cats:_____   Other:_____
• **Diet**: ☐Wet, ☐Dry; Brand/ Amt.:_____

Appetite	☐Normal, ☐↑, ☐↓
Weight	☐Normal, ☐↑, ☐↓; Past Wt.:_____ kg; Date:_____; Δ:_____
Thirst	☐Normal, ☐↑, ☐↓
Urination	☐Normal, ☐↑, ☐↓, ☐Blood, ☐Strain
Defecation	☐Normal, ☐↑, ☐↓, ☐Blood, ☐Strain, ☐Diarrhea, ☐Mucus
Discharge	☐No, ☐Yes; Onset/ Describe:
Cough/ Sneeze	☐No, ☐Yes; Onset/ Describe:
Vomit	☐No, ☐Yes; Onset/ Describe:
Respiration	☐Normal, ☐↑ Rate, ☐↑ Effort
Energy level	☐Normal, ☐Lethargic, ☐Exercise intolerance

• **Travel Hx**: ☐None, Other:_____
• **Exposure to**: ☐Standing water, ☐Wildlife, ☐Board/daycare, ☐Dog park, ☐Groomer
• **Adverse reactions to food/ meds**: ☐None, Other:_____
• Can give oral meds: ☐no ☐yes; Helpful Tricks:_____

Physical Exam:

T: *P:* *R:* *Wt.:* *BCS:* *Pain:* *CRT:*

☐*CV*: Regular rhythm, no murmur, normokinetic and synchronous pulses
☐*Resp*: Normal BV sounds/ effort, normal tracheal sounds/ palpation
☐*Attitude*: Bright, alert, and responsive
☐*Hydration/ Perfusion*: MM pink and moist with a CRT of 1-2 sec
☐*Eyes*: No abnormalities
☐*Nose*: No abnormalities
☐*Ears*: No abnormalities; ☐Debris (mild / mod / sev) (AU / AD / AS)
☐*Oral cavity*: No abnormalities; ☐Tarter (mild / mod/ sev); ☐Gingivitis
☐*Lymph nodes*: Small, symmetrical, smooth, and soft
☐*Abdomen*: Soft, non-painful, no fluid-wave, organomegaly, or masses
☐*Mammary Chain*: No abnormalities
☐*Penis/ Vulva*: No abnormalities
☐*Skin*: No alopecia, masses, erythema, other lesions, or ectoparasites
☐*Neuro*: No paresis, ataxia, or postural deficits, normal PLR and mentation
☐*MS*: Adequate and symmetrical muscling, no overt lameness
☐*Rectal*: No abnormalities, normal colored feces on glove

Labwork:

Other Diagnostics:
Blood Pressure:

Problem List:

Plan:

Case No._____

Patient	Age	Sex	Breed	Weigh
	DOB:	Mn / Mi Fs / Fi	Color:	k

Owner	Primary Veterinarian	Admit Date/ Time
Name: Phone:	Name: Phone:	Date: Time: AM / PM

• **Presenting Complaint**:_____

_____

_____

• **Medical Hx**:_____

_____

_____

• **When/ where obtained**:   Date:_____; ☐Breeder, ☐Shelter, Other:_____

Drug/ Suppl.	Amount	Dose (mg/kg)	Route	Frequency	Date Started

• **Vaccine status – Dog**: ☐Rab ☐Parv ☐Dist ☐Aden; ☐Para ☐Lep ☐Bord ☐Influ ☐Lyme
• **Vaccine status – Cat**: ☐Rab ☐Herp ☐Cali ☐Pan ☐FeLV[kittens]; ☐FIV ☐Chlam ☐Bord
• **Heartworm / Flea & Tick / Intestinal Parasites**:
   ◦ *Last Heartworm Test*: Date:_____, ☐IDK; Test Results: ☐Pos, ☐Neg, ☐IDK
   ◦ *Monthly heartworm preventative*: ☐no ☐yes, Product:_____
   ◦ *Monthly flea & tick preventative*: ☐no ☐yes, Product:_____
   ◦ *Monthly dewormer*: ☐no ☐yes, Product:_____
• **Surgical Hx**:   ☐Spay/Neuter; Date:_____; Other:_____
• **Environment**: ☐Indoor, ☐Outdoor, Time spent outdoors/ Other:_____
• **Housemates**: Dogs:_____ Cats:_____ Other:_____
• **Diet**: ☐Wet, ☐Dry; Brand/ Amt.:_____

Appetite	☐Normal, ☐↑, ☐↓
Weight	☐Normal, ☐↑, ☐↓; Past Wt.:_____ kg; Date:_____; Δ:_____
Thirst	☐Normal, ☐↑, ☐↓
Urination	☐Normal, ☐↑, ☐↓, ☐Blood, ☐Strain
Defecation	☐Normal, ☐↑, ☐↓, ☐Blood, ☐Strain, ☐Diarrhea, ☐Mucus
Discharge	☐No, ☐Yes; Onset/ Describe:
Cough/ Sneeze	☐No, ☐Yes; Onset/ Describe:
Vomit	☐No, ☐Yes; Onset/ Describe:
Respiration	☐Normal, ☐↑ Rate, ☐↑ Effort
Energy level	☐Normal, ☐Lethargic, ☐Exercise intolerance

• **Travel Hx**: ☐None, Other:_____
• **Exposure to**: ☐Standing water, ☐Wildlife, ☐Board/daycare, ☐Dog park, ☐Groomer
• **Adverse reactions to food/ meds**: ☐None, Other:_____
• Can give oral meds: ☐no ☐yes; Helpful Tricks:_____

Physical Exam:
T: P: R: Wt.:   BCS: Pain: CRT:

☐*CV*: Regular rhythm, no murmur, normokinetic and synchronous pulses
☐*Resp*: Normal BV sounds/ effort, normal tracheal sounds/ palpation
☐*Attitude*: Bright, alert, and responsive
☐*Hydration/ Perfusion*: MM pink and moist with a CRT of 1-2 sec
☐*Eyes*: No abnormalities
☐*Nose*: No abnormalities
☐*Ears*: No abnormalities; ☐Debris (mild / mod / sev) (AU / AD / AS)
☐*Oral cavity*: No abnormalities; ☐Tarter (mild / mod/ sev); ☐Gingivitis
☐*Lymph nodes*: Small, symmetrical, smooth, and soft
☐*Abdomen*: Soft, non-painful, no fluid-wave, organomegaly, or masses
☐*Mammary Chain*: No abnormalities
☐*Penis/ Vulva*: No abnormalities
☐*Skin*: No alopecia, masses, erythema, other lesions, or ectoparasites
☐*Neuro*: No paresis, ataxia, or postural deficits, normal PLR and mentation
☐*MS*: Adequate and symmetrical muscling, no overt lameness
☐*Rectal*: No abnormalities, normal colored feces on glove

Labwork:

Other Diagnostics:
Blood Pressure:

Problem List:

Plan:

Case No._____

Patient	Age	Sex	Breed	Weight
	DOB:	Mn / Mi Fs / Fi	Color:	kg

Owner	Primary Veterinarian	Admit Date/ Time
Name: Phone:	Name: Phone:	Date: Time: AM / PM

• **Presenting Complaint**:_____
_____
_____

• **Medical Hx**:_____
_____
_____

• **When/ where obtained**:   Date:_____; □Breeder, □Shelter, Other:_____

Drug/ Suppl.	Amount	Dose (mg/kg)	Route	Frequency	Date Started

• **Vaccine status – Dog**: □Rab □Parv □Dist □Aden; □Para □Lep □Bord □Influ □Lyme
• **Vaccine status – Cat**: □Rab □Herp □Cali □Pan □FeLV[kittens]; □FIV □Chlam □Bord
• **Heartworm / Flea & Tick / Intestinal Parasites**:
   ◦ *Last Heartworm Test*: Date:_____, □IDK; Test Results: □Pos, □Neg, □IDK
   ◦ *Monthly heartworm preventative*:   □no □yes, Product:_____
   ◦ *Monthly flea & tick preventative*:   □no □yes, Product:_____
   ◦ *Monthly dewormer*:   □no □yes, Product:_____
• **Surgical Hx**:   □Spay/Neuter; Date:_____; Other:_____
• **Environment**: □Indoor, □Outdoor, Time spent outdoors/ Other:_____
• **Housemates**: Dogs:_____ Cats:_____ Other:_____
• **Diet**: □Wet, □Dry; Brand/ Amt.:_____

Appetite	□Normal, □↑, □↓
Weight	□Normal, □↑, □↓; Past Wt.:_____ kg; Date:_____; Δ:_____
Thirst	□Normal, □↑, □↓
Urination	□Normal, □↑, □↓, □Blood, □Strain
Defecation	□Normal, □↑, □↓, □Blood, □Strain, □Diarrhea, □Mucus
Discharge	□No, □Yes; Onset/ Describe:
Cough/ Sneeze	□No, □Yes; Onset/ Describe:
Vomit	□No, □Yes; Onset/ Describe:
Respiration	□Normal, □↑ Rate, □↑ Effort
Energy level	□Normal, □Lethargic, □Exercise intolerance

• **Travel Hx**: □None, Other:_____
• **Exposure to**: □Standing water, □Wildlife, □Board/daycare, □Dog park, □Groomer
• **Adverse reactions to food/ meds**: □None, Other:_____
• Can give oral meds: □no □yes; Helpful Tricks:_____

Physical Exam:

T: *P:*   *R:*   *Wt.:*   *BCS:*   *Pain:*   *CRT:*

☐*CV*: Regular rhythm, no murmur, normokinetic and synchronous pulses
☐*Resp*: Normal BV sounds/ effort, normal tracheal sounds/ palpation
☐*Attitude*: Bright, alert, and responsive
☐*Hydration/ Perfusion*: MM pink and moist with a CRT of 1-2 sec
☐*Eyes*: No abnormalities
☐*Nose*: No abnormalities
☐*Ears*: No abnormalities; ☐Debris (mild / mod / sev) (AU / AD / AS)
☐*Oral cavity*: No abnormalities; ☐Tarter (mild / mod/ sev); ☐Gingivitis
☐*Lymph nodes*: Small, symmetrical, smooth, and soft
☐*Abdomen*: Soft, non-painful, no fluid-wave, organomegaly, or masses
☐*Mammary Chain*: No abnormalities
☐*Penis/ Vulva*: No abnormalities
☐*Skin*: No alopecia, masses, erythema, other lesions, or ectoparasites
☐*Neuro*: No paresis, ataxia, or postural deficits, normal PLR and mentation
☐*MS*: Adequate and symmetrical muscling, no overt lameness
☐*Rectal*: No abnormalities, normal colored feces on glove

Labwork:

Other Diagnostics:
Blood Pressure:

Problem List:

Plan:

Sources Cited:

1. *IRIS Staging of CKD.* © 2017 International Renal Interest Society (IRIS) Ltd.

2. Prittie, J. (2006). Optimal endpoints of resuscitation and early goal-directed therapy. *Journal of Veterinary Emergency and Critical Care, 16*(4), 329-339. doi:10.1111/j.1476-4431.2006.00160.x

3. *Shock Pathophysiology.* Edited by Elizabeth Thomovsky and Paula A. Johnson. © 2013 Vetstreet, Inc.

4. *Small Animal Clinical Diagnosis by Laboratory Methods*, Fifth Edition. Edited by Michael D. Willard and Harold Tvedten. © 2012 Saunders.

5. *Textbook of Small Animal Emergency*, First Edition. Edited by Kenneth J. Drobatz, Kate Hopper, Elizabeth Rozanski, and Deborah C. Silverstein. © 2019 John Wiley & Sons, Inc.

"Because you are alive, everything is possible."
- *Thich Nhat Hanh*

Physical Examination Findings at Each Stage of Shock

	DOG			CAT		
	Compensated Shock	Acute Decompensated Shock	Late Decompensated Shock	Compensated Shock	Acute Decompensated Shock	Late Decompensated Shock
Temp. (°F)	↓ (98–99)	↓↓ (96–98)	↓↓↓ (<96)	↓ (<97)	↓↓ (<95)	↓↓↓ (<90)
HR (bpm)	↑↑ (>180)	↑ (>150)	↓-to-N (<140)	↑↑↑ (>240) / ↓ (160–180)	↑↑ (>200) / ↓↓ (120–140)	↑ (>180) / ↓↓↓ (<120)
RR (rpm)	↑↑ (>50)	↑ (<50)	N-↑-Agonal	↑↑↑ (>60)	↑↑ (>60)	↑-to-Agonal
Mentation	QAR	Obtunded	Obtunded-to-Stupor	QAR	Obtunded	Obtunded-to-Stupor
MM color	Pale	Pale	Pale-to-Muddy	Pale	Pale-to-White	Pale-to-White
CRT (sec)	< 1	< 2	≥ 2	< 1	< 2	≥ 2
MAP (mm Hg)	↓-to-N (70–80)	↓ (50–70)	↓↓ (<60)	↓-to-N (80–90)	↓ (50–80)	↓↓ (<50)

- Source: 3

Endpoints of Resuscitation

Mentation	Normal
Heart Rate	Dog: 70–140; Cat: 140–180 (stressed: 180–220)
Blood Pressure	SAP >90 mmHg; MAP >60 mmHg
Lactate	< 2 mmol/L

- Source: 2

Fluid Therapy

Resuscitation	Hydration		
	Fluid Deficit / Dehydration	Maintenance	Ongoing Losses
Traditional "shock dose": ◦ **Dog = ¼ of 90 ml/kg** (over 15 min) ◦ **Cat = ¼ of 60 ml/kg** (over 15 min) Reevaluate based on endpoints of resuscitation.	• **Liters of dehydration = (kg) × (% dehydration)** • Subtract shock bolus volumes from fluid deficit. • Replace over 6–24 hour depending on patient. • Example: ◦ BW = 11 kg ◦ Estimated Dehydration = 7% ◦ Fluid deficit = (11)(0.07) = 0.77L = 770mL	• Traditional formulas: ◦ **Dog = 40–60 ml/kg/day** ◦ **Cat = 48–72 ml/kg/day** ◦ **Pediatric = 80–120 ml/kg/day** • Accounts for daily fluid losses from feces, skin, breathing, urine.	• Replace measured volumes of: ◦ Vomit ◦ Regurg. ◦ Diarrhea ◦ Saliva ◦ Blood loss ◦ Draining fluid

- Subcutaneous fluid dose (outpatient treatment of dehydration with mild clinical signs and normal tissue perfusion parameters): 10–30 mL/kg
- Source: 5

205

Reference Intervals

CBC:

- **RBC** (10^6/µl): *D-RI*: 5.5-8.5; *C-RI*: 5-10
- **PCV** (%): *D-RI*: 37-56; *C-RI*: 24-45
  - *Mild Anemia*: D30 –37; C20–26
  - *Moderate Anemia*: D20–29; C14–19
  - *Severe Anemia*: D13–19; C10–13
  - *Very Severe Anemia*: D<13; C<10
  - *Anemia of Chronic Disease*: D25–35; C20–25 (normocytic, normochromic)
- **HGB** (g/dl): *D-RI*: 10-20; *C-RI*: 8-15
- **MCV** (fL): *D-RI*: 60-77; *C-RI*: 39-55
- **MCHC** (g/dl): *D-RI*: 32-36; *C-RI*: 31-35
- **RETIC** (/µl): *D-Regen*: ≥60,000; *C-Regen*: ≥50,000 aggregate
- **WBC** (10^3/µl): *D-RI*: 6-17; *C-RI*: 5.5-19
  - *Leukemoid Reaction*: >50,000–100,000 /µl (without leukemia)
- **NEU** (10^3/µl): *D-RI*: 3-11.5; *C-RI*: 2.5-12.5
  - *Corticosteroid Response*: ~15,000–25,000 /µl (<40,000 /µl)
  - *Require Sepsis Monitoring*: <1,000–2,000 /µl
  - *Presumed Sepsis*: <500–1,000 /µl and febrile
  - *Suspend Chemotherapy with Myelosuppressive Agents*: <2,500 /µl
- **BAND** (/µl): *DC-RI*: 0-300
  - *Inflammatory Disease*: neutrophilia with a left shift >1,000 non-seg/µl
- **LYM** (10^3/µl): *D-RI*: 1-4.8; *C-RI*: 1.5-7
- **MONO** (/µl): *D-RI*: 150-1250; *C-RI*: 0-850
- **EOS** (/µl): *D-RI*: 100-1250; *C-RI*: 0-1500
- **BASO** (/µl): *DC-RI*: 0-150
- **PLT** (10^3/µl): *D-RI*: 200-500; *C-RI*: 300-800; *Greyhound Dogs*: ~150
  - *Risk of Spontaneous Thrombosis*: >1,000,000 /µl
  - *Risk of DIC*: >50,000 /µl and patient is spontaneously bleeding
  - *Risk of Spontaneous Bleed*: <30,000–50,000 /µl
  - *Top Differential is IMT*: <50,000 /µl
  - *Suspend Chemotherapy with Myelosuppressive Agents*: <50,000 /µl
  - *Normal Cavalier King Charles Spaniel & Norfolk Terrier*: <10,000 /µl
- **TS-Plasma** (g/dl): *DC-RI*: 6-8

Urinalysis:

- **USG** (GMS/1000): *Dog-RI*: ≥1.030; *Cat-RI*: ≥1.035
- **PH**: *DC-RI*: 6.0-7.0
- **Protein** (mg/dl): *D-RI*: 0-30 or trace with USG >1.012; *C-RI*: Neg
- **Glucose** (mg/dl): *DC-RI*: Neg
- **Ketones**: *DC-RI*: Neg
- **Bilirubin**: *D-RI*: Neg or trace with USG ≥1.030; *C-RI*: Neg
- **SSA** (protein): *D-RI*: 1+ with USG >1.012; *C-RI*: Neg
- **Acetest** (ketone): *DC-RI*: Neg
- **Ictotest** (bilirub): *D-RI*: Neg or trace with USG ≥1.030; *C-RI*: Neg
- **Casts** (/lpf): *DC-RI*: 0-2 hyaline or granular casts
- **WBC** (/hpf): *DC-RI*: <4
- **RBC** (/hpf): *DC-RI*: <5
- **Bacteria**: *DC-RI*: Neg in cysto sample
- **Cells** (/hpf): *DC-RI*: 0-2
- **Crystals**: *DC-RI*: None to Few
- **Urine Protein/Creatinine Ratio (U/PC)**:
  - *Non-proteinuric*:   D<0.2; C<0.2
  - *Borderline proteinuric*: D0.2-0.5; C0.2-0.4
  - *Proteinuric*:   D>0.5; C<0.4

Venous Blood Gas:

- **pH**:   *D-RI*: 7.32-7.40; *C-RI*: 7.28-7.41; (7.1<☘>7.6)
- **PCO2** (mm Hg): *D-RI*: 33-50;   *C-RI*: 33-45
- **HCO3** (mEq/L): *D-RI*: 18-26;   *C-RI*: 18-23

Arterial Blood Gas:

- **pH**:   *D-RI*: 7.36-7.44; *C-RI*: 7.36-7.44; (7.1<☘>7.6)
- **PCO2** (mm Hg): *D-RI*: 36-44;   *C-RI*: 28-32; (☘>70)
- **HCO3** (mEq/L): *D-RI*: 18-26;   *C-RI*: 17-22
- **PO2** (mm Hg): *D-RI*: ≈100;   *C-RI*: ≈100; (☘<60)

Serum Biochemistry:

- **Glucose** (mg/dl): *D-RI*: 60-135; *C-RI*: 65-131; (40<☕>1000)
  - ○ *Coma or Seizures*: <40; *Hyperosmotic diabetes with CNS dysfunction*: >1,000
- **Lactic Acid** (mg/dl): *D-RI*: 9.9-46.8; *C-RI*: 5.4-15.3
  - ○ Lactic Acid (mmol/L): *DC-RI*: 0.22-1.44; (☕>6.0; associated with a poor prognosis)
- **Cholesterol** (mg/dl): *D-RI*: 120-247; *C-RI*: 56-161
- **SDMA** (μg/dl): *DC-RI*: 0-14
- **BUN** (mg/dl): *D-RI*: 5-29; *C-RI*: 19-33
- **Creatinine** (mg/dl): *D-RI*: 0.3-2; *C-RI*: 0.8-1.8
- **Na** (mmol/l): *D-RI*: 139-147; *C-RI*: 144-155; (120<☕>170)
  - ○ *CNS signs*: <120 or >170 in dogs
- **K** (mmol/l): *D-RI*: 3.3-4.6; *C-RI*: 3.5-5.1; (2.5<☕>7.5)
  - ○ *Muscle weakness*: <2.5; *Cardiac conduction disturbances*: >7.5
- **Cl** (mEq/l): *D-RI*: 107-116; *C-RI*: 113-123
- **Na:K Ratio**: *Addison's suspect at* <27:1
- **Total Ca** (mg/dl): *D-RI*: 9.3-11.8; *C-RI*: 8.4-11.8; (7.0<☕>16)
  - ○ *Tetany*: <7.0; *Acute renal failure and cardiac toxicity*: >16
- **Ionized Ca** (mmol/L): *DC-RI*: 1.12-1.42
- **P** (mg/dl): *D-RI*: 2.9-6.2; *C-RI*: 3.8-7.5; (☕ <1.5)
  - ○ *Hemolysis, CNS signs*: <1.5
- **Ca×P Product** (mg/dL): Mineralization at >60
- **Mg** (mg/dl): *D-RI*: 1.7-2.1; *C-RI*: 1.7-2.3 (1<☕>10)
- **HCO3** (mmol/l): *D-RI*: 21-28; *C-RI*: 19-26 (☕ <12)
  - ○ *Suspect severe metabolic acidosis*: <12
- **AG** (mmol/l): *D-RI*: 10-18; *C-RI*: 12-19
- **OSM** (mOsm/kg): *D-RI*: 290-310; *C-RI*: 308-335
- **TP** (g/dl): *D-RI*: 5.7-7.8; *C-RI*: 6.1-7.7
- **Albumin** (g/dl): *D-RI*: 2.4-3.6; *C-RI*: 2.5-3.3; (☕ ≤1.5)
  - ○ *Severe hypoalbuminemia; at risk for major fluid shifts*: ≤1.5
- **Globulin** (g/dl): *D-RI*: 1.7-3.8; *C-RI*: 2.3-3.8
  - ○ *Severe hyperglobulinemia*: ≥5
- **Bilirubin** (mg/dl): *D-RI*: 0-0.8; *C-RI*: 0-0.6
  - ○ *Icteric plasma*: ≥1.5; *Icteric mucous membranes*: ≥3
- **ALT** (U/L): *D-RI*: 10-130; *C-RI*: 26-84
- **ALP** (U/L): *D-RI*: 24-147; *C-RI*: 20-109
- **GGT** (U/L): *D-RI*: 0-25; *C-RI*: 0-12

Other Diagnostics:

- **Systolic Blood Pressure** (mm Hg): *DC-RI*:
  - ○ *Hypo*: <80; *Normo*: 90–140; *Prehyper*: 140–159; *Hyper*: 160–179; *Severely Hyper*: ≥180
- **Mean Arterial Blood Pressure** (mm Hg): *DC-RI*: 60–100
- **Central Venous Pressure** (mm Hg): *DC-RI*: 3–8
- **SpO2** (Pulse Oximetry – hemoglobin saturation with oxygen) (%): *DC-RI*: ≥95
- **ETCO2** (Capnography – an estimate of PaCO2) (mm Hg): *DC-RI*: 35–45
- **BMBT** (min): *Normal platelet function in D*: 2.6 ± 0.5
- **D-Dimer** (μg/ml):
  - ○ <0.25 has a strong NPV to (more or less) rule out DIC
  - ○ >0.5 is characteristic for PTE in dogs (Se 100%; Sp 70%)
- **T4** (μg/dl): *D-RI*: 0.8-3.5; *C-RI*: 1-4
- **Cortisol** (μg/dl): *D-RI*: 1-6; *C-RI*: 1-5
  - ○ *Addison's suspect*: <2 (must perform ACTH-stimulation test)

- *Key: D – dog; C – cat; RI – reference interval; Regen – regenerative; Neg – negative; ☕ – danger values*
- *Helpful Equations:*
  - **RETIC** (/μl) = (RETIC[%]) × (RBC [10^6/μl])
  - **Corrected WBC count** = (NRBC × 100) / (NRBC + 100) [calculate if if nRBCs are >5]
  - **Corrected Total Serum Calcium** = tCa (mg/dl) – Alb (g/dl) + 3.5 [Calculate if ↓ alb]
  - **AG** = [Na + K] – [Cl + HCO3]
  - **OSM (Osmolality)** = 1.86(Na + K) + (BUN/2.8) + (Glucose/18) + 9
  - **Osmol Gap** = measured OSM – calculated OSM [>25 mOsm/kg = presence of unmeasured osmols]
  - *Sources*: 1, 4, 5; most CBC and serum biochemistry reference interval data are provided by the in-house Small Animal Clinical Pathology lab at the Texas A&M University Veterinary Medical Teaching Hospital

Emergency Drug Doses

Drug	Canine Dose	Feline Dose
Acepromazine	0.01–0.2 mg/kg, IV/ IM/ SC (max. 3 mg)	0.01–0.2 mg/kg, IV/ IM/ SC (max. 1 mg)
Apomorphine	0.03 mg/kg, IV (for emesis); 0.04 mg/kg, IM (for emesis); 0.02 mg/kg, SC (for emesis); 1.5–6 mg, in conjunctival sac (for emesis);	–
Atipamezole	3750 μg/m^2 BSA, IM (to reverse α2-agonists); 0.1 mg/kg, IV (to reverse α2-agonist in CPR)	Same
Atropine sulfate	0.04 mg/kg, IV/ IM/ IO (for CPR or atropine response test); 0.15–0.2 mg/kg, diluted 1:10 in saline or water, Intratrach	Same
Buprenorphine	0.005–0.03 mg/kg, IV/ IM/ SC, q6–12h; 0.12 mg/kg, Oral Transmucosal	0.01–0.03 mg/kg, IV/ IM, q6–8h; 0.03 mg/kg, Oral Transmucosal, q6–8h
Butorphanol	0.1–0.5 mg/kg, IV/ IM/ SC, q1–4h	0.1–0.5 mg/kg, IV/ IM/ SC, q1–4h
Butorphanol +Dexmedetomidine ± Ketamine	Butorphanol 0.4 mg/kg + Dexmedetomidine 0.005–0.01 mg/kg, mix in same syringe and give IM (if no evidence of cardiovascular disease)	Butorphanol 0.3 mg/kg + Dexmedetomidine 0.005–0.01 mg/kg ± Ketamine 3 mg/kg, mix in same syringe and give IM (duration of sedation is longer when ketamine is added)
Butorphanol +Midazolam +Other	Butorphanol 0.2 mg/kg, IV + Midazolam 0.2 mg/kg, IV + Alfaxalone 2 mg/kg, IV over 1 minute (provides excellent induction and recovery with minimal cardiopulmonary effects)	Butorphanol 0.4 mg/kg + Midazolam 0.4 mg/kg + Ketamine 3 mg/kg, mix in same syringe and give IM (provides good sedation for physiologically-compromised cats)
Calcium gluconate (10%)	1 mL/kg of 10% solution (which corresponds to 100 mg/kg of calcium gluconate), IV slowly over 10–20 min (for treatment of hyperkalemia with K$^+$ >8 mEq/L)	Same
Dexamethasone	0.07–0.14 mg/kg/day (anti-inflammatory), IV/ IM/ SC	Same
Dexmedetomidine	0.001–0.005 mg/kg, IV (or 125–375 μg/m^2 BSA, IV); 0.001–0.02 mg/kg, IM (or 165–500 μg/m^2 BSA, IM)	Same
Dextrose (50%)	0.5–1 mL/kg (0.25–0.5 g/kg), diluted 1:2 in sterile saline or water, IV slowly over 5 min (for treatment of hypoglycemia)	Same
Diazepam	0.5–2 mg/kg, IV/ Rectal/ Intranasal (for status epilepticus)	Same
Diphenhydramine	0.5–2 mg/kg, IV/ IM, q8–12h; 2–4 mg/kg, PO, q8–12h	Same
Epinephrine	0.01 mg/kg, IV/ IO, q3–5min in early CPR (low dose); 0.1 mg/kg, IV/ IO, q3–5min in prolonged CPR (high dose) * 1:1000=1 mg/mL; 1:10,000=0.1 mg/mL	Same
Flumazenil	0.01 mg/kg, IV/ IO, q1h as needed (to reverse benzodiazepines)	Same
Furosemide	1–4 mg/kg, IV/ IM/ SC, q1–2h	2–4 mg/kg, IV/ IM/ SC, q1–2h

Drug	Canine Dose	Feline Dose
Hydromorphone	0.05–0.2 mg/kg, IV/ IM/ SC, q2–4h (for analgesia)	0.05–0.1 mg/kg, IV/ IM/ SC, q2–6h
HES 6%	10–20 mL/kg, IV, given over 15–30 min (shock bolus)	5–10 mL/kg, IV, given over 15–30 min (shock bolus)
Hypertonic saline (7–7.5% NaCl)	4–5 mL/kg, IV, given over 5–10 min	3–4 mL/kg, IV, given over 5–10 min
Lidocaine[†]	2 mg/kg, IV, given over 2 min (for ventricular arrhythmia)	0.25–0.5 mg/kg, IV, given over 5 min (for ventricular arrhythmia)
Mannitol	0.5–1 g/kg, IV, given over 10–20 min, q6h	Same
Methadone	0.1–1 mg/kg, IV/ IM/ SC, q4–8h (for analgesia)	0.05–0.5 mg/kg, IV/ IM/ SC, q4–6h (for analgesia)
Midazolam	0.1–0.3 mg/kg, IV/ IM/ Intranasal (for status epilepticus)	Same
Morphine	0.5–1 mg/kg, IV/ IM/ SC, given over 2 min, q2h (for analgesia)	0.05–0.4 mg/kg, IM/ SC, q3h (for analgesia)
Naloxone	0.01–0.04 mg/kg, IV/ IM/ SC/ IO (to reverse opioid)	Same
Packed RBCs	10 mL/kg, IV (1 mL/kg to raise PCV 1%)	Same
Plasma	6–20 mL/kg, IV, PRN for coagulopathy	Same
Prednisolone	0.5–1 mg/kg/day (anti-inflammatory), IV/ PO	Same
Procainamide	2 mg/kg, IV, given over 3–5 min, up to a total dose of 20 mg/kg (for atrial or ventricular arrhythmia)	–
Propofol	2–6 mg/kg, IV slowly to effect	Same
Terbutaline	–	0.01 mg/kg, IV/ IM/ SC, q4h (for asthma)
Whole blood	10–20 mL/kg, IV (2 mL/kg to raise PCV 1%)	Same
Xylazine	–	0.4–1.1 mg/kg, IV/ IM/ SC (for emesis)

† *Clinically-significant ventricular tachycardia*: ≥4 ventricular premature complexes consecutively at a rate of ≥160 bpm in dogs (≥240 bpm in cats)
- Sources: 3, 8, 11

45427131R00115